Basic Guide to Medical Emergencies in the Dental Practice

BASIC GUIDE TO MEDICAL EMERGENCIES IN THE DENTAL PRACTICE

Second Edition

Phil Jevon

RN, BSc (Hons), PGCE
Medical Education, Walsall Healthcare NHS Trust
Walsall, UK
Honorary Clinical Lecturer (Medicine), University of Birmingham
Birmingham, UK

Consulting Editors

Celia Strickland, BDS Dental Practitioner, Staffordshire, UK

Tessa Meese, Lead DCP Tutor, Health Education, West Midlands, UK; Dental Nurse Manager, Birmingham Dental Hospital, Birmingham, UK; Editor-in-Chief, Dental Nursing

Jagtar Singh Pooni, BSc (Hons), MRCP (England), FRCA, Consultant in Anaesthesia & Intensive Care Medicine, New Cross Hospital, Wolverhampton, UK

WILEY Blackwell

This edition first published 2014
© 2010 by Phil Jevon
© 2014 by John Wiley & Sons, Ltd

Registered office: John Wiley & Sons, Ltd, The Atrium, Southern Gate, Chichester, West Sussex, PO19 8SQ, UK

Editorial offices: 9600 Garsington Road, Oxford, OX4 2DQ, UK
The Atrium, Southern Gate, Chichester, West Sussex, PO19 8SQ, UK
111 River Street, Hoboken, NJ 07030-5774, USA

For details of our global editorial offices, for customer services and for information about how to apply for permission to reuse the copyright material in this book please see our website at www.wiley.com/wiley-blackwell

Library of Congress Cataloging-in-Publication Data
Jevon, Philip, author.
  Basic guide to medical emergencies in the dental practice / Phil Jevon; consulting editors, Celia Strickland, Tessa Meese, Jagtar Singh Pooni. — Second edition.
      p. ; cm.
  Includes bibliographical references and index.
  ISBN 978-1-118-68883-0 (pbk.)
  I. Strickland, Celia, editor. II. Meese, Tessa, editor. III. Pooni,
J. S. (Jagtar Singh), editor. IV. Title.
  [DNLM: 1. Dental Care—methods. 2. Emergency Treatment—methods.
  3. Emergencies. WU 105]
  RK51.5
  617.6'026—dc23

                                                                    2013043841

A catalogue record for this book is available from the British Library.

Wiley also publishes its books in a variety of electronic formats. Some content that appears in print may not be available in electronic books.

Cover image: courtesy of Phil Jevon
Cover design by Workhaus

Set in 10/12.5 pt Sabon LT Std by Aptara Inc., New Delhi, India

Printed in the UK

Contents

Foreword   ix

Acknowledgements   x

About the companion website   xi

1 An overview of the management of medical emergencies and
   resuscitation in the dental practice   1
   Introduction   1
   Concept of the chain of survival   2
   Incidence of medical emergencies in dental practice   3
   General dental council guidelines on medical emergencies   4
   Resuscitation Council (UK) quality standards   5
   ABCDE assessment of the sick patient   6
   Medical risk assessment in general dental practice   7
   Principles of safer handling during cardiopulmonary resuscitation   8
   Procedure for calling 999 for an ambulance   10
   Importance of human factors and teamwork   11
   Conclusion   13
   References   13

2 Resuscitation equipment in the dental practice   15
   Introduction   15
   Recommended minimum resuscitation equipment in
      the dental practice   16
   Checking resuscitation equipment and drugs   20
   Checking resuscitation equipment following use   22
   Care, handling and storage of oxygen cylinders   23
   Conclusion   25
   References   25

3 ABCDE: Recognition and treatment of the acutely ill patient   26
   Introduction   26
   Clinical signs of acute illness and deterioration   27
   The ABCDE approach   27
   General principles of the ABCDE approach   28
   The ABCDE approach to the sick patient   28
   Principles of pulse oximetry   34
   Procedure for administering oxygen to the acutely ill patient   38
   Procedure for recording blood pressure   41

Medical emergencies in the dental practice poster   44
Conclusion   46
References   46

4 Respiratory disorders   48
Introduction   48
Management of acute asthma attack   49
Management of hyperventilation   55
Management of exacerbation of chronic obstructive pulmonary disease   56
Procedure for using an inhaler   57
Procedure for using a spacer device   61
Conclusion   64
References   64

5 Cardiovascular disorders   66
Introduction   66
Management of angina   67
Management of myocardial infarction   69
Management of palpitations   73
Management of syncope   74
Conclusion   76
References   77

6 Endocrine disorders   78
Introduction   78
Management of hypoglycaemia   78
Procedure for blood glucose measurement using a glucometer 83
Management of adrenal insufficiency   85
Conclusion   86
References   86

7 Neurological disorders   88
Introduction   88
Management of a generalised tonic–clonic seizure   88
Management of stroke   93
Management of altered level of consciousness   96
Procedure for placing a patient in the recovery position   97
Spinal injury   101
Conclusion   102
References   102

8 Anaphylaxis   104
Introduction   104
Definition   105
Incidence   105
Pathophysiology   105
Causes   106

Clinical features and diagnosis   107
Treatment   109
Risk assessment   113
Conclusion   114
References   115

9 Cardiopulmonary resuscitation in the dental practice   117
Introduction   117
Resuscitation Council (UK) automated external defibrillation algorithm 118
Procedure for cardiopulmonary resuscitation in the dental chair 118
Procedure for performing chest compressions   126
Conclusion   129
References   130

10 Airway management and ventilation   131
Introduction   131
Causes of airway obstruction   132
Recognition of airway obstruction   132
Simple techniques to open and clear the airway   133
Use of oropharyngeal airway   135
Principles of ventilation   138
Treatment of foreign body airway obstruction   147
Conclusion   150
References   150

11 Automated external defibrillation   152
Introduction   152
Ventricular fibrillation   153
Physiology of defibrillation   153
Factors affecting successful defibrillation   154
Safety issues and defibrillation   155
Procedure for automated external defibrillation   155
Conclusion   158
References   158

12 Paediatric emergencies   160
Introduction   160
ABCDE assessment of a sick child   161
Principles of paediatric resuscitation   162
Placing a child into the recovery position   170
Management of foreign body airway obstruction   170
Conclusion   173
References   173

13 An overview of emergency drugs in the dental practice   175
Introduction   175
Adrenaline   176

Aspirin   179
Glucagon   180
Glyceryl trinitrate spray   181
Midazolam   182
Oral glucose solution/tablets/gel/powder   185
Salbutamol inhaler   185
Conclusion   187
References   187

14 Principles of first aid in the dental practice   189
    Introduction   189
    Priorities of first aid   190
    Responsibilities when providing first aid   190
    Assessment of the casualty   190
    Wounds and bleeding   195
    Minor burns and scalds   200
    Poisoning, stings and bites   200
    Importance of record keeping   202
    Summary   203
    References   203

15 Professional, ethical and legal issues   204
    Introduction   204
    The scope of a dental professional's accountability   205
    The fifth sphere of accountability   217
    Legal requirements for consent and acting in a patient's
      best interests   218
    Duty of confidence owed to patients by dental professionals   226
    Conclusion   231
    References   232

Index   235

Foreword

It is a pleasure to write a foreword for this text which covers a range of medical emergencies in dental practice. It is well laid out, easy to follow and a very useful resource for all members of the dental team and especially helpful for dentists, dental therapists and hygienists and dental nurses. The General Dental Council's Standards for the Dental Team states we should follow the guidance on medical emergencies and training updates issued by the Resuscitation Council (UK), this text conveniently pulls much of that information together into a very readable form.

We never know when these skills may be required. Although we may do everything we can to try to prevent a medical emergency, we have to be vigilant and prepared when looking after our patients. You can be confident in the content of this book as it follows national guidelines and forms a very convenient reference text.

I would encourage all members of the dental team to read this work and also to dip into it periodically for useful reminders. Students and qualified professional groups will find it very useful.

Professor Philip J. Lumley
BDS, FDSRCPS, FDSRCS, MDentSc, PhD
University of Birmingham School of Dentistry

Acknowledgements

I would like to thank Steve Webb and Mandeep Dhanda, together with the dental staff at Walsall Healthcare NHS Trust, for their help with the images.

I would like to thank Richard Griffith for kindly updating his "Professional, Ethical and Legal Issues" chapter.

About the companion website

This book is accompanied by a companion website:

www.wiley.com\go\jevon\medicalemergencies

The website includes:

- 50 interactive Multiple-Choice Questions
- Powerpoints of all figures from the book for downloading

Chapter 1

An overview of the management of medical emergencies and resuscitation in the dental practice

INTRODUCTION

Every dental practice has a duty of care to ensure that an effective and safe service is provided for its patients (Jevon, 2012). The satisfactory performance in a medical emergency or in a resuscitation attempt in the dental practice has wide-ranging implications in terms of resuscitation equipment, resuscitation training, standards of care, clinical governance, risk management and clinical audit (Jevon, 2009).

The Resuscitation Council (UK) (2013) has updated its standards for clinical practice and training in resuscitation for dental practitioners and dental care professionals in general dental practice. All members of the dental team need to be aware of what their role would be in the event of a medical emergency and should be trained appropriately with regular practice sessions (Greenwood, 2009).

The aim of this chapter is to provide an overview of the management of medical emergencies and resuscitation in the dental practice.

LEARNING OUTCOMES

At the end of the chapter the reader will be able to:
- Discuss the concept of the chain of survival
- Discuss the incidence of medical emergencies in the dental practice
- Outline the General Dental Council guidelines on medical emergencies
- Summarise the Resuscitation Council (UK) standards
- Discuss the principles of safer handling during cardiopulmonary resuscitation (CPR)
- Outline the procedure for calling 999 for an ambulance
- Discuss the importance of human factors and teamwork in a medical emergency

Basic Guide to Medical Emergencies in the Dental Practice, Second Edition. Phil Jevon.
© 2014 John Wiley & Sons, Ltd. Published 2014 by John Wiley & Sons, Ltd.
Companion website: www.wiley.com\go\jevon\medicalemergencies

CONCEPT OF THE CHAIN OF SURVIVAL

Survival from cardiac arrest relies on a sequence of time-sensitive interventions (Nolan *et al.*, 2010). The concept of the original chain of survival emphasised that each time-sensitive intervention must be optimised in order to maximise the chance of survival: a chain is only as strong as its weakest link (Cummins *et al.*, 1991).

The chain of survival (Figure 1.1) stresses the importance of recognising critical illness and/or angina and preventing cardiac arrest (both in and out of hospital) and post-resuscitation care (Nolan *et al.*, 2006):

- *Early recognition and call for help to prevent cardiac arrest:* this link stresses the importance of recognising patients at risk of cardiac arrest, dialling 999 for the emergency services and providing effective treatment to hopefully prevent cardiac arrest (Nolan *et al.*, 2010); patients sustaining an out-of-hospital cardiac arrest usually display warning symptoms for a significant duration before the event (Müller *et al.*, 2006).
- *Early CPR to buy time* and *early defibrillation to restart the heart:* the two central links in the chain stress the importance of linking CPR and defibrillation as essential components of early resuscitation in an attempt to restore life. Early CPR can double or even triple the chances of a patient surviving an out-of-hospital ventricular fibrillation (shockable rhythm) induced cardiac arrest (Holmberg *et al.*, 1998, 2001; Waalewijn *et al.*, 2001).
- *Post-resuscitation care to restore quality of life:* the priority is to preserve cerebral and myocardial function and to restore quality of life (Nolan *et al.*, 2010).

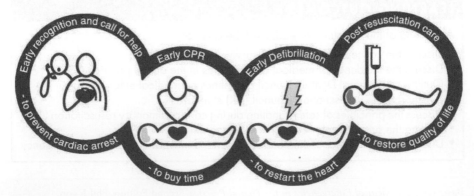

Figure 1.1 Chain of survival. *Source:* Laerdal Medical Ltd, Orpington, Kent, UK. Reproduced with permission.

INCIDENCE OF MEDICAL EMERGENCIES IN DENTAL PRACTICE

The incidence of medical emergencies in dental practice is very low. Medical emergencies occur in hospital dental practice more frequently, but in similar proportions to that found in general dental practice (Atherton *et al.*, 2000). With the elderly population in dental practices increasing, medical emergencies in the dental practice will undoubtedly occur (Dym, 2008).

A literature search for published surveys on the incidence of medical emergencies and resuscitation in the dental practice found the following.

Survey of dental practitioners in Australia

A postal questionnaire survey of 1250 general dental practitioners undertaken in Australia (Chapman, 1997) found that:

- one in seven (14%) had had to resuscitate a patient;
- the most common medical emergencies encountered were adverse reactions to local anaesthetics, grand mal seizures, angina and hypoglycaemia.

Survey of dentists in England

A survey of dentists (Girdler and Smith, 1999) (300 responded) in England found that over a 12-month period they had encountered:

- vasovagal syncope (63%) – 596 patients affected;
- angina (12%) – 53 patients affected;
- hypoglycaemia (10%) – 54 patients affected;
- epileptic fit (10%) – 42 patients affected;
- choking (5%) – 27 patients affected;
- asthma (5%) – 20 patients affected;
- cardiac arrest (0.3%) – 1 patient affected.

Survey of dental practitioners in a UK university dental hospital

Atherton *et al.* (2000) assessed the frequency of medical emergencies by undertaking a survey of clinical staff (dentists, hygienists, nurses and radiographers) at a university dental hospital. The researchers found that:

- fainting was the commonest event;
- other medical emergency events were experienced with an average frequency of 1.8 events per year;
- highest frequency of emergencies were reported by staff in oral surgery.

Survey of dentists in New Zealand

A total of 199 dentists responded to a postal survey undertaken by Broadbent and Thomson (2001) in New Zealand, with the following findings:

- Medical emergencies had occurred in 129 practices (65.2%) within the previous 10 years (mean – 2.0 events per 10,000 patients treated under local analgesia, other forms of pain control or sedation);
- Vasovagal events were the most common emergencies occurring in 121 (61.1%) practices within the previous year (mean 6.9 events per 10,000 patients treated under local analgesia, other forms of pain control or sedation).

Survey of dental staff in Ohio

A survey of dental staff in Ohio (Kandray *et al.*, 2007) found that 5% had performed CPR on a patient in their dental surgery.

Survey of dentists in Germany

A survey of 620 dentists in Germany (Müller *et al.*, 2008) found that in a 12-month period:

- 57% had encountered up to 3 emergencies;
- 36% had encountered up to 10 emergencies;
- Vasovagal episode was the most common reported emergency – average 2 per dentist;
- 42 dentists (7%) had encountered an epileptic fit;
- 24 dentists (4%) had encountered an asthma attack;
- 5 dentists (0.8%) had encountered choking;
- 7 dentists (1.1%) had encountered anaphylaxis;
- 2 dentists (0.3%) had encountered a cardiopulmonary arrest.

GENERAL DENTAL COUNCIL GUIDELINES ON MEDICAL EMERGENCIES

Standards for the Dental team (General Dental Council, 2013) emphasises that all dental professionals are responsible for putting patients' interests first, and acting to protect them. Central to this responsibility is the need for dental professionals to ensure that they are able to deal with medical emergencies that may arise in their practice. Such emergencies are, fortunately, a rare occurrence, but it is important to recognise that a medical emergency could happen at any time and that all members of the dental team need to know their role in the event of one occurring.

The General Dental Council, in its publication *Principles of Dental Team Working* (General Dental Council, 2006), states that the person who employs, manages or leads a team in a dental practice should ensure that:

- There are arrangements for at least two people available to deal with medical emergencies when treatment is planned to take place;
- All members of staff, not just the registered team members, know their role if a patient collapses or there is another kind of medical emergency;
- All members of staff who might be involved in dealing with a medical emergency are trained and prepared to deal with such an emergency at any time;
- Members of the team practice together regularly in a simulated emergency so they know exactly what to do.

Maintaining the knowledge and competence to deal with medical emergencies is an important aspect of all dental professionals continuing professional development (General Dental Council, 2006). The above guidance has been endorsed by the Resuscitation Council (UK) (2013).

RESUSCITATION COUNCIL (UK) QUALITY STANDARDS

The Resuscitation Council (UK)'s Quality standards for cardiopulmonary resuscitation practice and training: primary dental care (2013) provides guidance and recommendations concerning the management of a cardiac arrest in the dental practice.

Topics covered include medical risk assessment, resuscitation procedures and the use of resuscitation equipment in the dental practice in general dental practice. It also includes topics such as staff training, patient transfer and post-resuscitation/emergency care.

The key recommendations in the statement are that:

- Every dental practice should have a procedure in place for medical risk assessment of their patients;
- Specific resuscitation equipment should be immediately available in every dental practice (this should be standardised throughout the United Kingdom);
- Every clinical area should have immediate access to an automated external defibrillator (AED);

- Dental practitioners and dental care professionals should receive training in CPR, including basic airway management and the use of an AED, with annual updates;
- Regular simulated emergency scenarios should take place in the dental practice;
- Dental practices should have a protocol in place for calling medical assistance in an emergency (this will usually be calling 999 for an ambulance);
- All medical emergencies should be audited.

For further information, access the Resuscitation Council (UK)'s website http://www.resus.org.uk/pages/QSCPR_PrimaryDentalCare.htm accessed 4 December 2013).

'A patient could collapse on any premises at any time, whether they have received treatment or not. It is therefore essential that ALL registrants are trained in dealing with medical emergencies, including resuscitation, and possess up to date evidence of capability'. General Dental Council 'Scope of Practice' 2013

ABCDE ASSESSMENT OF THE SICK PATIENT

Many people who suffer an out-of-hospital cardiac arrest display warning symptoms for a significant duration before collapse (Müller *et al.*, 2006). These symptoms could include:

- chest pain;
- dyspnoea (breathlessness);
- nausea/vomiting;
- dizziness/syncope. (Müller *et al.*, 2006)

The Resuscitation Council (UK) (2012) recommends the ABCDE approach to assess the sick patient (see Chapter 3). All dental professionals should be familiar with the approach because, not only will it help them to recognise the warning symptoms which many people exhibit prior to sudden cardiac arrest, but also it will help to establish whether the patient is sick or not. The logical and systematic ABCDE approach to assessing the sick patient incorporates:

- airway;
- breathing;
- circulation;
- disability;
- exposure.

When assessing the patient, a complete initial assessment should be undertaken, identifying and treating life-threatening problems first, before moving on to the next part of assessment. The effectiveness of treatment/intervention should be evaluated and regular reassessment undertaken. The need to call for an ambulance should be recognised and other members of the multidiscipli-nary team should be utilised as appropriate so that patient assessment, instiga-tion of appropriate monitoring and interventions can be undertaken.

MEDICAL RISK ASSESSMENT IN GENERAL DENTAL PRACTICE

Although any patient could experience a medical emergency in general prac-tice, certain patients will be at higher risk. It is therefore important to identify these patients by undertaking medical and medication histories. The dental practitioner can then take measures to reduce the chance of a problem arising in dental practice.

History taking

Medical and medication histories should be obtained by the dental practi-tioner and should not be delegated to another member of the dental team; if a patient completes a health questionnaire it is only acceptable if augmented by a verbal history taken by the dental practitioner (Resuscitation Council (UK), 2012). For some patients, it may be necessary to modify the planned treatment or even refer them for treatment in hospital.

Risk stratification scoring system

A risk stratification scoring system, e.g. the American Society of Anaesthe-siologists' classification, should be used routinely by the dental practitioner when assessing a patient for dental treatment, as it may help to identify those patients who are at greater risk of a medical emergency during dental treat-ment (Resuscitation Council (UK), 2012). It should trigger hospital referral for treatment if a certain level of risk is attained. It has been suggested that a risk stratification could be incorporated into the routine medical history questionnaire so that all patients are risk assessed (Resuscitation Council (UK), 2012).

Up-to-date patient details

It is recommended to update the patient's medical and medication histories on a regular basis (at least annually) or more frequently as required; it may be necessary to liaise with the patient's general practitioner (Resuscitation Coun-cil (UK), 2012).

Existing medical problem

Patients with certain existing medical problems are more likely to suffer a medical emergency in the dental surgery:

- *Angina:* if a patient has frequent episodes of angina following exertion or suffers from angina that is easily provoked, he or she may experience an episode of angina in the dental practice. If the patient suffers from angina episodes caused by anxiety or stress, he may benefit from being prescribed an oral anxiolytic drug, e.g. diazepam, before dental treatment. *Note:* prolonged drug treatment may lead to dependence (British Medical Association and The Royal Pharmaceutical Society, 2013. The patient should be considered at higher risk if he or she has unstable angina, angina episodes at night or has had a recent admission to hospital with angina. For these patients, in-hospital treatment may be prudent (Resuscitation Council (UK), 2012).
- *Asthma:* an asthmatic patient is more likely to have a severe asthma attack in the dental practice if he or she has had a previous near-fatal asthmatic episode, if he has been admitted to the emergency department with asthma in the previous 12 months, or if he has been prescribed three or more classes of medication, or if he regularly requires beta-2 agonist therapy (British Thoracic Society, 2008).
- *Epilepsy:* the patient will usually be able to provide the dental practitioner with a good indication of how well his condition is controlled. There is a greater risk of having a fit in the dental practice if his fits are poorly controlled or if his medications have recently been altered. It would be prudent to ascertain the timings of, and precipitating factors for, the patient's last three fits (Resuscitation Council (UK), 2012).
- *Diabetes:* a patient with Type 1 diabetes (on insulin) is more likely become hypoglycaemic in the dental practice than a patient with Type 2 diabetes (diet or tablet controlled); patients whose diabetes is poorly controlled or who have poor awareness of their hypoglycaemic episodes are more likely to develop hypoglycaemia (Resuscitation Council (UK), 2012).
- *Allergies:* it is important to ascertain whether the patient has any known allergies, particularly to local anaesthetic, antibiotics or latex. If the patient has a severe latex allergy, use latex-free gloves; he should either be treated in a hospital environment or in a latex-free dental environment where appropriate resuscitation facilities are at hand (Resuscitation Council (UK), 2012).

PRINCIPLES OF SAFER HANDLING DURING CARDIOPULMONARY RESUSCITATION

The Resuscitation Council (UK), in its publication *Guidance for Safer Handling during Resuscitation in Healthcare Settings* (2009), has issued guidelines concerning safer handling during CPR. Although specifically aimed at hospital staff, the guidelines can be adapted for use when performing CPR in the dental practice. An overview will now be provided. Although the use of slide sheets is recommended when moving the patient, these are not usually available in the dental practice.

Cardiac arrest on the floor

- If the patient has collapsed on the floor, e.g. in the waiting room, perform CPR on the floor. If the area has restricted access, consider sliding the patient across the floor.
- Ventilation: kneel behind the patient's head ensuring the knees are shoulder-width apart, rest back to sit on the heels and lean forwards from the hips towards the patient's face.
- Chest compressions: kneel at the side of the patient, level with his chest, and adopt a high kneeling position with the knees shoulder-width apart; position the shoulders directly over the patient's sternum and keeping the arms straight compress the chest ensuring the force for compressions results from flexing the hips.

Cardiac arrest in the dental chair

- Remove any environmental hazards, e.g. mouthwash, dental instrument tray.
- Lower the chair into a horizontal position.
- Ventilation: to use the mask device, ideally sit on the dentist's stool at the head end of the chair. The person squeezing the bag should stand with their feet in a walk/stand position facing the patient; avoid prolonged static postures.
- Chest compressions: ensure the chair is at a height which places the patient between the knee and mid-thigh of the person performing chest compressions; stand at the side of the chair with the feet shoulder-width apart, position the shoulders directly over the patient's sternum and, keeping the arms straight, compress the chest, ensuring the force for compressions results from flexing the hips.

Cardiac arrest in a chair in the waiting room

- Lowering the patient to the floor: with two colleagues, slide the patient on to the floor; ideally a third person should support the patient's head during the procedure.

Cardiac arrest in the toilet

- Ensure the toilet door is kept open and access maintained.
- Lowering the patient to the floor: with two colleagues, slide the patient on to the floor; ideally a third person should support the patient's head during the procedure.

PROCEDURE FOR CALLING 999 FOR AN AMBULANCE

There are many emergency situations in the dental practice which will require an ambulance to be called, e.g. chest pain, difficulty with breathing, anaphylaxis and cardiopulmonary arrest. When calling 999 for an ambulance, the following is a suggested procedure:

- If available, obtain the 'when dialling 999 information card' that will have the dental practice's address, telephone number and any specific instructions or guidelines if the practice is difficult to find. Reading from this card will make it easier for the person calling 999 for an ambulance and will help minimise the risk of incorrect information being given.
- Lift the telephone receiver or switch the phone on and dial 999 (when using a telephone in a dental practice it is usually necessary to access an outside line first, e.g. by pressing a specific key or pressing 9).
- When the telephone operator answers, he or she will ask which emergency service you require. Tell the operator that you need an ambulance and you will then be connected to the ambulance service. (It is important to remember that 999 (or 112) is used for other emergencies as well such as the fire service, police, mountain rescue, coastguard.)
- Once connected to the ambulance service, the ambulance control officer (Figure 1.2) will ask you where you would like the ambulance to come to, the telephone number of the phone you are calling from and details of the

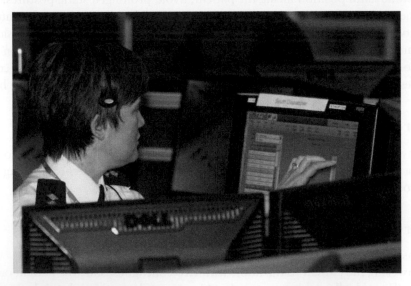

Figure 1.2 Ambulance control centre. *Source*: West Midlands Ambulance Service. Reproduced with permission.

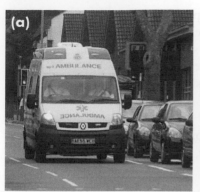
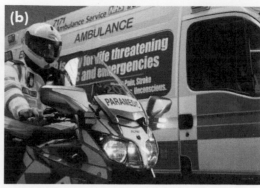

Figure 1.3 (a) Ambulance. Reproduced with kind permission from West Midlands Ambulance Service. **(b)** Paramedic on a motorcycle. *Source*: West Midlands Ambulance Service. Reproduced with permission.

emergency. Give accurate details of the address or location where help is needed. If there is a recognisable landmark, e.g. famous shop nearby, this information will be helpful. An ambulance or paramedic on a motorcycle will be dispatched (Figures 1.3a and 1.3b).
- If appropriate, stay on the line and continue to listen to important advice provided by the ambulance control officer.
- Confirm with the senior dental practitioner that an ambulance has been called.
- Note the time the 999 call was made.
- If possible, ask someone to wait outside the dental practice to attract the attention of the ambulance when it draws near (a patient may be willing to do this).

It is important to:

- stay calm;
- listen carefully to any questions the operator may ask;
- speak slowly and clearly; do not shout.

IMPORTANCE OF HUMAN FACTORS AND TEAMWORK

When managing a medical emergency, technical skills, e.g. administration of oxygen or using an AED are important if the patient's outcome is to be optimized. However, there is another group of skills, that are also important, that are becoming increasingly recognised in medicine – human factors or non-technical skills (Resuscitation Council (UK), 2011). These human factors can be defined as the cognitive, social and personal resource skills that complement technical skills and contribute to safe and efficient task performance and these skills affect the individual's personal performance (Resuscitation Council (UK), 2012).

Deficiencies in the requisite human factors are a common cause of adverse incidents associated with medical emergencies (Norris and Lockey, 2012). Human factors play a major role in these shortcomings and that the medical performance depends on the quality of leadership and team-structuring (Huniziker *et al.*, 2010).

To help minimise the risk of human factors adversely affecting the performance of the team in a medical emergency, the Resuscitation Council (UK, 2011) recommends the following:

- **Situational awareness:** during a medical emergency, it is important for all team members to have a common understanding of current events (shared situational awareness)
- **Decision making:** the team leader (usually the senior dentist) should be making decisions and communicating these clearly and unambiguously to the team members
- **Team working, including team leadership:** clear team leadership is associated with more efficient co-operation in the team and with better task performance; leaders who participated "hands-on" in the emergency were less likely to be efficient leaders, and team performance usually suffers (Hunziker *et al.*, 2010). Attributes of a good team leader are listed in Box 1.1
- **Task management:** co-ordination of tasks undertaken during an emergency ensuring they are done, e.g. calling 999 for an ambulance

---

Box 1.1   Attributes of a good team leader

- Knows all team members by name
- Understands each team member's capability
- Accepts role of team leader
- Delegates tasks appropriately
- knowledgeable and credible
- Remains calm and focused in an emergency
- Keeps team focused and controls distractions
- Communicates effectively (both giving instructions and listening)
- Empathic towards the whole team
- Assertive and authoritative when appropriate
- Understanding/tolerant towards hesitancy or nervousness in an emergency
- Good situational awareness
- Following emergency, thanks team and supports both staff and relatives as required
- Completes documentation and ensures an adequate handover

Source: Resuscitation Council (UK) (2011).

CONCLUSION

Dental practitioners have a duty of care to ensure that an effective and safe service is provided for their patients. This chapter has provided an overview of the management of medical emergencies and resuscitation with specific reference to the standards for clinical practice and training in medical emergencies and resuscitation for dental practitioners and dental care professionals in general dental practice.

REFERENCES

Atherton G, Pemberton M, Thornhill M (2000) Medical emergencies: the experience of staff of a UK dental teaching hospital. *British Dental Journal*; 12;188(6):320–324.

British Medical Association & the Royal Pharmaceutical Society of Great Britain (2013) *British National Formulary 65*. Royal Pharmaceutical Society, London.

British Thoracic Society (2008) *British Guideline on the Management of Asthma*. British Thoracic Society, London.

Broadbent J, Thomson W (2001) The readiness of New Zealand general dental practitioners for medical emergencies. *New Zealand Dental Journal*; 97(429):82–86.

Chapman P (1997) Medical emergencies in dental practice and choice of emergency drugs and equipment: a survey of Australian dentists. *Australian Dental Journal*; 42(2):103–108.

Cummins R, Ornato J, Thies W, Pepe P (1991) Improving survival from sudden cardiac arrest: the "chain of survival" concept. A statement for health professionals from the Advanced Cardiac Life Support Subcommittee and the Emergency Cardiac Care Committee, American Heart Association. *Circulation*; 83:1832–1847.

Dym H (2008) Preparing the dental office for medical emergencies. *Dental Clinics of North America*; 52(3):605–608.

General Dental Council (2013) *Standards for the Dental Team*. GDC, London.

General Dental Council (2006) *Principles of Dental Team Working*. GDC, London.

Girdler N, Smith D (1999) Prevalence of emergency events in British dental practice and emergency management skills of British dentists. *Resuscitation*; 41:159–167.

Greenwood M (2009) Medical emergencies in dental practice: 1. The drug box, equipment and general approach. *Dental Update*; 36:202–211.

Holmberg M, Holmberg S, Herlitz J (2001) Factors modifying the effect of bystander cardiopulmonary resuscitation on survival in out-of-hospital cardiac arrest patients in Sweden. *European Heart Journal*; 22:511–519.

Holmberg M, Holmberg S, Herlitz J, Gardelov B (1998) Survival after cardiac arrest outside hospital in Sweden. *Swedish Cardiac Arrest Registry Resuscitation*; 36:29–36.

Hunziker S, Tschan F, Semmer N *et al.* (2010) Human factors in resuscitation: lessons learned from simulator studies. *Journal of Emergencies, Trauma and Shock*; 3(4):389–394.

Jevon P (2009) *Medical Emergencies in the Dental Practice*, Wiley-Blackwell, Oxford.

Jevon P (2012) Updated guidance on medical emergencies and resuscitation in the dental practice. *British Dental Journal*; 212(1):41–43.

Kandray D, Pieren J, Benner R (2007) Attitudes of Ohio dentists and dental hygien-ists on the use of automated external defibrillators. *Journal of Dental Education*; 71(4):480–486.

Müller D, Agrawal R, Arntz H (2006) How sudden is sudden cardiac death? *Circula-tion*; 114:1146–1150.

Müller M, Hänsel M, Stehr S *et al.* (2008) A state-wide survey of medical emergency management in dental practices: incidence of emergencies and training experience. *Emergency Medicine Journal*; 25:296–300.

Nolan J, Soar J, Zideman DA *et al.* (2010) European Resuscitation Council Guidelines for Resuscitation 2010 Section 1. *Resuscitation*; 81:1219–1276.

Nolan J, Soar J, Eikeland H (2006) Image in resuscitation: the chain of survival. *Resus-citation*; 71:270–271.

Norris E, Lockey A (2012) Human factors in resuscitation teaching *Resuscitation*; 83(4):423–427.

Resuscitation Council (UK) (2011) *Advanced Life Support*, 6th Edn. Resuscitation Council (UK), London

Resuscitation Council (UK) (2012) *Medical emergencies and resuscitation standards for clinical practice and training for dental practitioners and dental care profession-als in general dental practice*, Resuscitation Council (UK), London.

Resuscitation Council (UK) (2013) *Quality standards for cardiopulmonary resuscita-tion practice and training*: primary dental care, Resuscitation Council (UK), London www.resus.org.uk (accessed 4 December 2013).

Waalewijn RA, Tijssen JG, Koster RW (2001) Bystander initiated actions in out-of-hospital cardiopulmonary resuscitation: results from the Amsterdam Resuscitation Study (ARREST). *Resuscitation*; 50:273—9.

Chapter 2

Resuscitation equipment in the dental practice

INTRODUCTION

It is recommended that resuscitation equipment for any medical emergency or cardiopulmonary arrest should be standardised throughout dental practices in the United Kingdom (Resuscitation Council (UK), 2013). Successful resuscitation partly relies on the availability and correct functioning of resuscitation equipment (Dyson and Smith, 2002). The Resuscitation Council (UK) (2013) has made recommendations on the provision and use of resuscitation equipment in the dental practice. Other additional equipment will be required if the dental practice undertakes sedation.

All dental staff who may be involved in dealing with a cardiopulmonary arrest or a medical emergency must be prepared to deal with it (General Dental Council, 2006). Procedures must therefore be in place to ensure that the recommended resuscitation equipment is immediately available and in working order. In addition, dental staff must know where it is stored within their working area and how to use it safely and effectively (Greenwood, 2009; Resuscitation Council (UK), 2013).

The aim of this chapter is to discuss the provision of resuscitation equipment in the dental practice.

LEARNING OUTCOMES

At the end of this chapter the reader will be able to:

- List the recommended minimum resuscitation equipment in the dental practice
- Discuss the routine checking of emergency equipment
- Discuss the checking of emergency equipment following use
- Discuss the care, handling and storage of oxygen cylinders

Basic Guide to Medical Emergencies in the Dental Practice, Second Edition. Phil Jevon.
© 2014 John Wiley & Sons, Ltd. Published 2014 by John Wiley & Sons, Ltd.
Companion website: www.wiley.com\go\jevon\medicalemergencies

RECOMMENDED MINIMUM RESUSCITATION EQUIPMENT IN THE DENTAL PRACTICE

The Resuscitation Council (UK) (2012, 2013) recommends the following minimum equipment for the management of a medical emergency or cardiopulmonary arrest in the dental practice.

Airway equipment

- Set of oropharyngeal airways sizes 1, 2, 3 and 4 (Figure 2.1).
- Portable suction device with appropriate suction catheters and tubing (Figure 2.2), e.g. Yankauer Sucker.

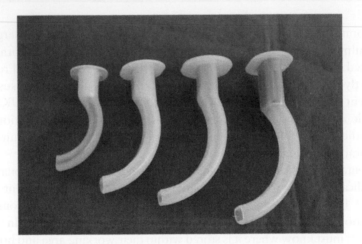

Figure 2.1 Oropharyngeal airways.

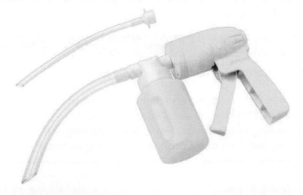

Figure 2.2 Portable suction device. *Source*: Timesco, Basildon, UK. Reproduced with permission.

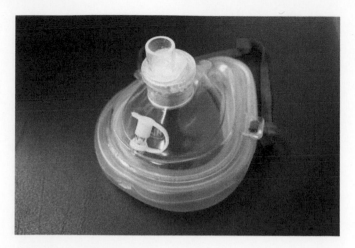

Figure 2.3 Pocket mask with oxygen port.

Breathing equipment

- Pocket mask with oxygen port (Figure 2.3).
- Self-inflating resuscitation bag with oxygen reservoir and tubing (Figure 2.4) (if local staff have been trained to use it).
- Selection of well-fitting adult and child face masks for attaching to the self-inflating bag.
- Oxygen face mask with oxygen reservoir and tubing (Figure 2.5).

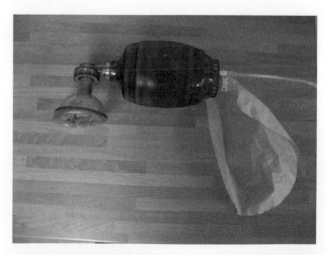

Figure 2.4 Self-inflating resuscitation bag with oxygen reservoir and tubing.

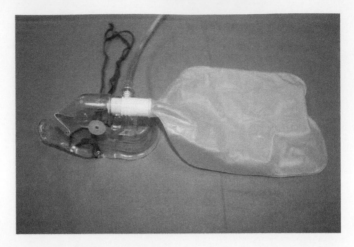

Figure 2.5 Oxygen face mask with tubing.

- Portable oxygen cylinder (D size) with pressure reduction valve and flowmeter (Figure 2.6).
- Oxygen cylinder key (if appropriate).
- 'Spacer device' for inhaled bronchodilator.

Circulation equipment

- Automated external defibrillator (AED) (Figure 2.7) (with defibrillation electrodes, pair of heavy duty scissors and a razor).
- Sterile syringes — e.g. 1 or 2 ml syringes for drawing up adrenaline 1:1000 solution from an ampoule.

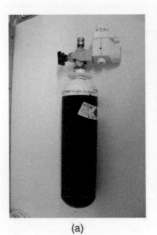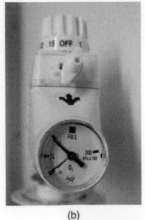

(a)   (b)

Figure 2.6 (a) Portable oxygen cylinder (D size) with **(b)** pressure reduction valve and flowmeter.

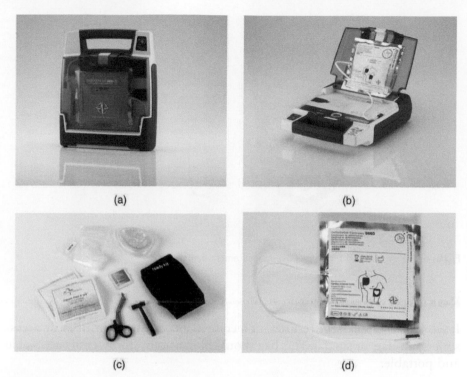

(a)   (b)

(c)   (d)

Figure 2.7 Automated external defibrillator (AED) **(a)** closed, **(b)** open, with **(c)** defibrillation electrodes, a pair of heavy-duty scissors and a razor, and **(d)** adult pads.

- Sterile needles — size 23 gauge (blue) (suitable for most age groups) and size 21 gauge (green) for larger adults (Department of Health, 2013).

Drugs

- Glyceryl trinitrate (GTN) spray (400 μg/dose).
- Salbutamol aerosol inhaler (100 μg/actuation).
- Adrenaline injection (1:1000, 1 mg/ml).
- Aspirin dispersible 300 mg.
- Glucagon injection 1 mg.
- Oral glucose solution/tablets/gel/powder.
- Midazolam 10 mg (buccal or injection).

(*Source*: British Medical Association & Royal Pharmaceutical Society of Great Britain, 2013)

Additional items

- Automated blood glucose measurement device (Figure 2.8).
- Gloves.

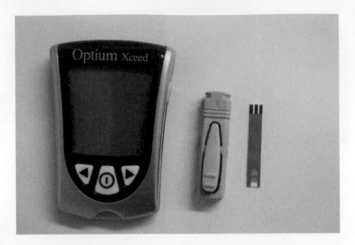

Figure 2.8 Automated blood glucose measurement device.

Resuscitation bag

It would be helpful if the resuscitation equipment was stored in an easily accessible 'grab-bag' or similar. This bag should be spacious, sturdy, easily accessible and portable.

CHECKING RESUSCITATION EQUIPMENT AND DRUGS

Each individual dental practice is responsible for checking its resuscitation equipment (Resuscitation Council (UK), 2013). Named individuals should be nominated to check equipment which should be carried out at least weekly and the checking process audited (Greenwood, 2009). This weekly check is also recommended by the Resuscitation Council (UK) (2013).

Equipment inventory

Having an equipment inventory is helpful as it will assist the checking of the resuscitation equipment.

Drugs

All drugs should be stored together, ideally in a purpose-designed container (Greenwood, 2009). Expiry dates of the drugs should be checked and there should be a planned replacement programme in place (Resuscitation Council (UK), 2013).

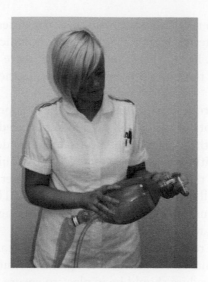

Figure 2.9 Checking self-inflating resuscitation bag.

Although the reclassification of midazolam as a 'Schedule 3' controlled drug requires certain legal processes, this does not include requirements for safe custody, i.e. locked cupboard, nor the need to keep a midazolam controlled drug register (Resuscitation Council (UK), 2012). Some healthcare institutions are encouraging such practices as part of their own health and safety protocols but there is no legal obligation to do so (Jevon, 2012).

Self-inflating bag

The self-inflating bag should be checked to ensure that there are no leaks (Figure 2.9) and that the rim of the face mask is adequately inflated. Older reusable devices should be particularly carefully checked because they are prone to perishing. Ideally, they should be replaced with new single-use (and latex-free) devices.

Defibrillator

If the dental practice has a defibrillator, it should be checked following the manufacturer's recommendations.

Automated external defibrillators

Most AEDs perform self-checks on a daily basis and will alert staff if a problem is identified, e.g. if the battery requires replacement. Generally, the only checks required to be undertaken by dental staff are that the device is 'rescue ready' and that the defibrillation electrodes are not out of date.

The 'AED is fine to use' indicator varies between different makes and models. In the AED depicted in Figure 2.7, a green light indicates that the defibrillator is 'rescue ready'. If the AED is indicating that there is a problem (usually by an audible bleep), this should be investigated and the problem rectified as soon as possible.

Defibrillation electrodes usually have a shelf life of approximately 18 months to 2 years. Once out of date, they will need to be replaced. A procedure should be in place to ensure that replacement electrodes are ordered in advance.

Most AEDs use lithium batteries that do not require recharging. Once installed in the AED, the battery will last a specified period of time, typically up to 5 years (this will be reduced if the AED is used). There should be a procedure in place to ensure that a new battery is ordered, again in advance of the current one requiring to be replaced.

Some AEDs use a rechargeable battery: it is important to ensure that the battery is charged and recharged following the manufacturer's recommendations. Again, a procedure should be in place to ensure that this happens.

Some AEDs need to be kept on charge: it is important to ensure that the AED is kept on charge following the manufacturer's recommendations. Again, a procedure should be in place to ensure that this happens.

> Most AEDs do not need to be switched on for checking — doing this will actually run down the battery

Manual defibrillators

Some dental practices have a manual defibrillator. It is usually necessary for this to remain plugged into the mains to ensure that the battery is fully charged in the event of use. It is important to ensure that the appropriate defibrillation gel pads and electrodes are available. It is common practice for manual defibrillators to be maintained and serviced by the electro-biomedical engineers (EBME) department at the local hospital.

Single use and latex free

Ideally, all emergency equipment should be single use and latex free (Greenwood, 2009; Resuscitation Council (UK), 2013).

CHECKING RESUSCITATION EQUIPMENT FOLLOWING USE

Checking of resuscitation equipment following use should be a specifically delegated responsibility. As well as the routine checks identified above, any disposable equipment used should be replaced and reusable equipment, e.g. self-inflating bag, cleaned following local infection control procedures and manufacturer's recommendations. Any difficulties with equipment encountered during resuscitation should be documented and reported to relevant personnel.

CARE, HANDLING AND STORAGE OF OXYGEN CYLINDERS

Portable oxygen cylinders are black with white shoulders (Marcovitch, 2005). There are many different types of portable cylinders available. A commonly used one is featured in Figure 2.6. This cylinder has:

- A regulator integrated with the cylinder valve
- A gauge that shows 'live' contents at all times, even when the cylinder is turned off
- Simple on—off handwheel (no tools needed)
- Click-stop flow control knob showing flow in litres per minute, ranging from 1 to 15 l/min
- Sufficient capacity to last approximately 30 minutes at highest flow rate of 15 l/min

Source: BOC Medical (2009)

When using an oxygen cylinder, always follow the manufacturer's recommendations. Before using the oxygen cylinder in Figure 2.6:

- If necessary, remove the protective cap
- Attach the oxygen tubing and mask to the fir tree outlet (the oxygen outlet) of the cylinder
- Ensure the flow control knob on the top of the cylinder is set at '0'
- Open the valve slowly by turning the grey or black handwheel anti-clockwise two revolutions
- Turn the flow control knob clockwise to select the required flow rate. At each full 'click' a different flow rate setting will be revealed in the 'window' of the knob. The correct flow rate setting must be fully visible in the window
- Select flow rate as per training received
- Check for a flow of gas through the mask prior to use

Source: Jevon (2009) BOC Medical (2009)

After using the oxygen cylinder in Figure 2.6:

- Turn off cylinder using the grey or black handwheel by turning it clockwise
- Remove tubing and mask from the fir tree outlet and allow residual oxygen in the regulator to vent

- Turn flow control knob to '0'
- Check the cylinder contents gauge to ensure adequate supply for next administration

Source: Jevon (2009), BOC Medical (2009)

The MHRA (2008) has issued guidance on the care and handling of oxygen cylinders and their regulators. It recommends that healthcare staff should:

- Be fully trained in the use of oxygen cylinders
- Be aware of all the related risks such as fire and manual handling
- Carry out full checks on oxygen cylinders and their regulators prior to each use, ensuring that they contain enough oxygen for the required therapy.
- Check the label on the oxygen cylinder ensuring it is not out-of-date
- Ensure their hands are clean before handling an oxygen cylinder; there is a risk of combustion from oils and grease. It is also important to ensure their hands are adequately dried after the use of alcohol gel.
- Ensure that the oxygen cylinder outlet and oxygen regulator inlet are clean before attaching a regulator
- Always open the cylinder slowly and check for leaks. Close cylinder valves when not in use.
- Handle oxygen cylinders with care. If the cylinder is dropped or knocked in use it must be checked before further use; cylinders with integral valves should be returned to the supplier; separate regulators should be sent to the service department for inspection.

The MHRA (2008) recommends that oxygen cylinders should be stored in a secure area that is well ventilated, clean and dry, as well as being free from any sources of ignition such as patients/staff smoking or machinery.

BOC Medical (2009) advises that it is important to:

- Keep the oxygen cylinder away from naked flames and sources of heat. Oxygen is a non-flammable gas, but it does strongly support combustion
- Ensure the oxygen cylinders are stored in a safe and secure area where they cannot fall over and cause injury
- Ensure the oxygen cylinder is stored in a well-ventilated area
- Never use excessive force when opening or closing the cylinder using the grey or black handwheel
- Not paint the cylinders as all labels and markings must remain clearly visible
- Refrain from using oil or grease (or any oil-based products which includes hand creams) in the vicinity of the oxygen cylinder. High velocity oxygen and oil/grease could cause spontaneous combustion

Source: BOC Medical (2009)

Defective oxygen cylinders should be reported to the Defective Medicines Reporting Centre (DMRC) and defective detachable regulators to the Adverse Incident Centre (AIC), both at the MHRA (www.mhra.gov.uk).

CONCLUSION

This chapter has detailed what resuscitation equipment should be immediately available in the event of a medical emergency or cardiopulmonary arrest. Suggestions have been made regarding the storage, checking and maintenance of this equipment.

REFERENCES

BOC Medical (2009) *Instructions for Using a CD Oxygen Cylinder,* www.bochealthcare. co.uk (accessed 14 October 2009).

British Medical Association & Royal Pharmaceutical Society of Great Britain (2013) *BNF 66.* BMJ Publishing, London.

Department of Health (2013) *Immunisation Against Infectious Diseases* Department of Health, London https://www.wp.dh.gov.uk/immunisation/files/2012/09/Green-Book-updated-280113_test.pdf (accessed 16 February 2013).

Dyson E, Smith G (2002) Common faults in resuscitation equipment — guidelines for checking equipment and drugs used in adult cardiopulmonary resuscitation. *Resuscitation*; 55(2):137–149.

General Dental Council (2006) *Principles of Dental Team Working.* GDC, London.

Greenwood M (2009) Medical emergencies in dental practice: 1. The drug box, equipment and general approach. *Dental Update*; 36:202–211.

Jevon P (2009) Practical procedures: administering oxygen. *Dental Nursing*; 5(4):615–617.

Jevon P (2012) Buccolam(®) (buccal midazolam): a review of its use for the treatment of prolonged acute convulsive seizures in the dental practice. *British Dental Journal*; 213(2):81–82.

Marcovitch H (2005) *Black's Medical Dictionary.* Black, London.

MHRA (2008) *Top Tips on Care and Handling of Oxygen Cylinders and Their Regulators*, MHRA, London.

Resuscitation Council (UK) (2012) *Medical Emergencies and Resuscitation Standards for Clinical Practice and Training for Dental Practitioners and Dental Care Professionals in General Dental Practice*, Resuscitation Council (UK), London.

Resuscitation Council (UK) (2013) Minimum equipment list for cardiopulmonary resuscitation: primary dental care, Resuscitation Council (UK), London, www.resus. org.uk (accessed 5 December 2013).

Chapter 3

ABCDE: Recognition and treatment of the acutely ill patient

INTRODUCTION

It is important to have a systematic approach to an acutely ill patient and to remain calm (Greenwood, 2009). The Resuscitation Council (UK) (2012) recommends undertaking a systematic clinical assessment following the ABCDE approach: pre-empting a medical emergency would allow appropriate help, e.g. ambulance, to be called, hopefully before the patient deteriorates or collapses. As well as monitoring the patient's vital signs, e.g. respiratory rate, pulse and blood pressure it is also important to be alert to the presence of chest pain (see Chapter 6), a common pre-cardiac arrest symptom (Resuscitation Council (UK), 2012).

The aim of this chapter is to understand the principles of recognition of the acute ill patient following the ABCDE approach.

LEARNING OUTCOMES

At the end of this chapter the reader will be able to:

- List the clinical signs of acute illness and deterioration
- Describe the ABCDE approach
- List the general principles of the ABCDE approach
- Describe the ABCDE approach to the sick patient
- Discuss the principles of pulse oximetry
- Describe the procedure for administering emergency oxygen
- Outline the procedure for recording the blood pressure
- Describe the use of the *Medical Emergencies in the Dental Practice* poster

Basic Guide to Medical Emergencies in the Dental Practice, Second Edition. Phil Jevon.
© 2014 John Wiley & Sons, Ltd. Published 2014 by John Wiley & Sons, Ltd.
Companion website: www.wiley.com\go\jevon\medicalemergencies

CLINICAL SIGNS OF ACUTE ILLNESS AND DETERIORATION

The clinical signs of acute illness and deterioration are usually similar regardless of the underlying cause, because they reflect compromise of the respiratory, cardiovascular and neurological functions (Nolan *et al.*, 2005). These clinical signs are commonly:

- Tachypnoea (respiratory rate > 20/min): a particularly important indicator of an at-risk patient (Goldhill *et al.*, 1999) and is the most common abnormality found in acute illness (Goldhill and McNarry, 2004);
- Tachycardia (heart rate > 100 beats per minute);
- Hypotension (usually a systolic blood pressure < 90mmHg);
- Altered consciousness level (e.g. lethargy, confusion, restlessness or falling level of consciousness) (Resuscitation Council (UK), 2012; Jevon and Ewens, 2012).

The identification of the clinical signs of acute illness (together with the patient's history, examination and appropriate investigations) is central to objectively identifying patients who are acutely ill or deteriorating (Buist *et al.*, 1999). However, these clinical signs of deterioration are often subtle and can go unnoticed. It is therefore important to assess the patient following the systematic ABCDE approach.

THE ABCDE APPROACH

The Resuscitation Council (UK) (2012) has issued guidance on the recognition and treatment of the sick patient following the logical and systematic ABCDE approach:

- Airway;
- Breathing;
- Circulation;
- Disability;
- Exposure.

When assessing the patient, undertake a complete initial assessment, identifying and treating life-threatening problems first, before moving on to the next part of assessment. The effectiveness of treatment/intervention should be evaluated, and regular reassessment undertaken. The need to call for an ambulance should be recognised and other members of the multidisciplinary team should be utilised as appropriate so that patient assessment, instigation of appropriate monitoring and interventions can be undertaken simultaneously.

RECOGNITION AND TREATMENT OF THE ACUTELY ILL PATIENT

Irrespective of their training, experience and expertise in clinical assessment and treatment, all dental professionals can follow the ABCDE approach; clinical skills, knowledge, expertise and local circumstances will determine what aspects of the assessment and treatment are undertaken.

GENERAL PRINCIPLES OF THE ABCDE APPROACH

The general principles of the ABCDE approach to assessing the acutely ill patient are as follows:

- The ABCDE approach should be followed when both assessing and treating the patient.
- Life-threatening problems, once identified, should be treated before moving on to the next part of the assessment.
- If there is further deterioration, reassessment should be performed, starting with the airway.
- The effects of any treatment administered should be evaluated.
- The need for extra help, e.g. calling 999 for an ambulance, should be considered.
- All the members of the dental team should be involved, allowing essential tasks such as collecting emergency equipment and oxygen or calling 999 for an ambulance to be undertaken simultaneously.
- Effective organisation and communication within the dental team are paramount.
- The initial aim of treatment is to keep the patient alive, prevent deterioration and ideally achieve clinical improvement; hopefully this will buy time while awaiting expert help and more definitive treatment.
- The ABCDE approach can be used by dental professionals irrespective of their training, expertise and experience in clinical assessment or treatment; individual experience and training will determine which aspects of assessment are undertaken and which treatments are administered.
- Basic interventions, e.g. laying the patient flat or administering oxygen, are often all that are required.

Source: Resuscitation Council (UK) (2012)

THE ABCDE APPROACH TO THE SICK PATIENT

Safety
Ensure the environment is safe and free of hazards and follow infection control guidelines, e.g. wash hands, put on gloves if necessary.

Communication

Talk to the patient and evaluate his response: a normal response, indicates he has a clear airway, is breathing and has adequate cerebral perfusion; the inability to complete sentences could indicate extreme respiratory distress. An inappropriate response or no response could indicate an acute life-threatening physiological disturbance (Gwinnutt, 2006), e.g. inability to complete sentences in one breath is a severe adverse sign in a patient having an asthmatic attack (British Thoracic Society, 2008).

Patient's general appearance

Note the patient's general appearance, his colour and whether he appears content and relaxed or distressed and anxious.

Senior help

It is important to call for help at a very early stage – this includes anything from other members of the dental team to calling for an ambulance (Greenwood, 2009). Request help from the senior dental practitioner. During the assessment process, consider whether it is necessary to call 999 for an ambulance.

Oxygen, emergency equipment/drugs

Ask a colleague to fetch the oxygen and other emergency equipment/drugs if required.

Monitoring devices

If one is available, attach a pulse oximeter (see principles of pulse oximetry section later) (Resuscitation Council (UK), 2012).

Airway

Assessment of airway

During the assessment of the airway, it is important to quickly establish if it is obstructed and treat it effectively. Look, listen and feel for the signs of airway obstruction. Partial airway obstruction will result in noisy breathing.

- *Gurgling:* indicates the presence of fluid, e.g. secretions or vomit, in the mouth or upper airway; usually seen in a patient with altered level of consciousness who is having difficulty or is unable to clear his own airway.
- *Snoring:* indicates that the pharynx is being partially obstructed by the tongue; usually seen in a patient with altered level of consciousness lying in a supine position.
- *Stridor:* high-pitched sound during inspiration, indicating partial upper airway obstruction; usually due to either a foreign body or laryngeal oedema.

RECOGNITION AND TREATMENT
OF THE ACUTELY ILL PATIENT

- *Wheeze:* noisy musical whistling type sound due to the turbulent flow of air through narrowed bronchi and bronchioles, more pronounced on expiration; causes include asthma and chronic obstructive pulmonary disorder (COPD).
- Complete airway obstruction can be detected by no air movement at the patient's mouth and nose. Paradoxical chest and abdominal movements ('see-saw' movement of the chest) may be observed and, if not rapidly treated, central cyanosis will develop (late sign of airway obstruction).

Treatment of airway obstruction

Airway obstruction is a medical emergency. If untreated, it can lead to hypoxia/hypoxaemia (low oxygen levels in the blood), which can damage the brain, kidneys and heart; cardiac arrest and even death could ensue (Resuscitation Council (UK), 2011).

If the patient has airway obstruction, whether partial or complete, treat the underlying cause if possible. In most situations, simple interventions are sufficient to clear the airway. For example:

- Perform head tilt, chin lift to open the airway in an unconscious patient (see Chapter 10).
- Suction the pharynx if there is blood or vomit in it.
- Consider inserting an oropharyngeal airway to help keep a patent airway in an unconscious patient (see Chapter 10).
- Perform back slaps and abdominal thrusts as necessary if there is foreign body airway obstruction (see Chapter 10).
- Administer oxygen 15 l/min via a non-rebreathe mask (Figure 3.1) (see Chapter 10) (Jevon and Ewens, 2012).

Breathing

Assessment of breathing

During the assessment of breathing, it is important to quickly diagnose and treat any life-threatening breathing problems, e.g. acute asthma (Resuscitation Council (UK), 2012). Follow the familiar 'look, listen and feel' approach to assess breathing:

- *Count the respiratory rate:* normal respiratory rate is 12–20 beats per minute (Resuscitation Council (UK), 2012). Tachypnoea (fast respiratory rate) is usually the first sign that the patient has respiratory distress. It is an indicator of illness, that the patient may deteriorate and that medical help is required (Resuscitation Council (UK), 2012). Bradypnoea (slow respiratory rate) is an ominous sign and could indicate imminent respiratory arrest; causes include drugs, e.g. opiates, and fatigue.

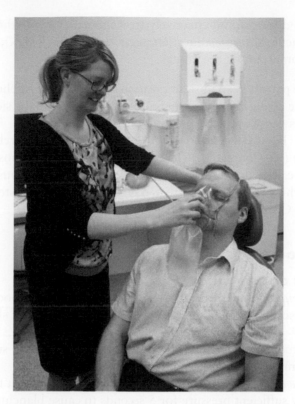

Figure 3.1 Administering high concentration of oxygen via a non-rebreathe mask.

- *Evaluate chest movement:* chest movement should be symmetrical; unilateral chest movement suggests unilateral pathology, e.g. pneumothorax, pneumonia, pleural effusion.
- *Evaluate the depth of breathing:* only marked degrees of hyperventilation and hypoventilation can be detected; hyperventilation may be seen if the patient is having a panic attack (Ford *et al.*, 2005).
- *Note the oxygen saturation (SaO₂) reading (if available):* the normal reading is usually 97–100%. A low SaO_2 could indicate respiratory distress or compromise.
- *Listen to the breathing:* normal breathing is quiet. Rattling airway noises indicate the presence of airway secretions, usually due to the patient being unable to cough sufficiently or unable to take a deep breath in. The presence of stridor or wheeze indicates partial, but significant, airway obstruction (see *Assessment of airway* section above).

Treatment of compromised breathing
If the patient has compromised breathing it is paramount to provide prompt effective treatment. In addition, during the initial assessment of breathing, it

is essential to diagnose and effectively treat immediately life-threatening conditions, e.g. acute severe asthma (Resuscitation Council (UK), 2012). If the patient has compromised breathing:

- Position the patient in an upright position to help maximise chest movement; if he is in the dental chair, he may find it helpful to sit on the side of the chair with his legs down and feet touching the floor.
- Administer high concentration of oxygen via a non-rebreathe mask (Figure 3.1) (see Chapter 10) (Jevon and Ewens, 2012); If possible treat the underlying cause. In the dental practice the most likely cause of compromised breathing that could be treated is asthma, i.e. administer beta agonist inhaler (see Chapter 4).

Circulation

Assessment of circulation

- *Count the pulse (radial or carotid):* a weak pulse suggests a poor cardiac output. In a vasovagal attack, the pulse is slow; in anaphylactic shock the pulse is fast.
- *Check the colour and temperature of the hands and fingers:* signs of cardiovascular compromise include cool and pale peripheries.
- *Measure the capillary refill time (CRT):* holding a fingertip at the level of the heart, apply sufficient pressure for 5 seconds to cause blanching of the skin, and then release (Figure 3.2). Normal CRT is less than 2 seconds; a prolonged CRT could indicate poor peripheral perfusion, though other causes can include cool ambient temperature, poor lighting and old age (Resuscitation Council (UK), 2012). A prolonged capillary refill time may be seen in anaphylaxis.

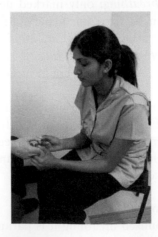

Figure 3.2 Measuring capillary refill time.

- *Measure the blood pressure:* a systolic BP <90 mm Hg suggests shock.
- *Establish if the patient has chest pain:* central crushing chest pain is suggestive of a heart attack (see Chapter 5).

Treatment of a problem with circulation

The treatment of a problem with circulation will depend on the cause:

- *Low blood pressure due to a vasovagal episode or simple faint:* lay the patient flat with the legs raised (often, no other treatment is required) (see Chapter 5).
- *Anaphylactic shock:* lay the patient flat with the legs raised (unless this compromises breathing), administer high concentration of oxygen and administer adrenaline, while a colleague calls 999 for an ambulance.
- *Chest pain:* sit patient upright; treatment could include GTN spray, aspirin and high inspired concentration oxygen; it will usually be necessary to dial 999 for an ambulance.
- Administer high concentration of oxygen via a non-rebreathe mask if necessary (Figure 3.1) (see Chapter 10) (Jevon and Ewens, 2012).

Disability

Assessment of disability

To assess disability (central nervous system function):

- *Evaluate the patient's level of consciousness:* use the AVPU method and assign the patient as being A (alert), V (responds to a vocal stimulus), P (responds to a painful stimulus) or U (unresponsive to all stimuli) (Resuscitation Council (UK), 2012) (Figure 3.3). Causes of altered level of consciousness include hypoxia, cerebral hypoperfusion due to low blood pressure, and recent administration of sedative or analgesic medications.
- *Examine the pupils:* compare size, equality and reaction to light of each pupil. Recent injection of an illicit drug (opiate) can cause pinpoint pupils.
- *Check the blood glucose:* if the patient has altered level of consciousness, check the blood glucose to exclude hypoglycaemia (see Chapter 6).
- *Check the patient's medication history:* is there a reversible drug-induced cause of altered level of consciousness?

> **A**lert
> **R**esponds to **V**oice
> Responds to **P**ain
> **U**nresponsive

Figure 3.3 AVPU: scale for assessing level of consciousness.

Treatment of altered level of consciousness

- Review Airway Breathing Circulation to exclude hypoxia or low blood pressure as a cause of altered level of consciousness.
- Consider placing the patient in the lateral position to help protect the airway, particularly if unresponsive to all stimuli.
- Consider administering high concentration of oxygen via a non-rebreathe mask (Figure 3.1) (see Chapter 3) (Jevon and Ewens, 2012).
- If hypoglycaemia is suspected/confirmed, administer appropriate treatment to raise blood glucose levels (see Chapter 6).
- Consider the need to call 999 for an ambulance.

Exposure

In order to assess and treat the patient properly, it may be necessary to loosen or remove some of his clothes; his dignity should be respected and heat loss minimised (Resuscitation Council (UK), 2011). If anaphylaxis is suspected, examine the skin for urticaria and angioedema (skin swelling).

PRINCIPLES OF PULSE OXIMETRY

Some dental practices (usually only those that administer sedation) will have access to a pulse oximeter (Figure 3.4). It will therefore be helpful to discuss the principles of pulse oximetry and oxygen saturation monitoring.

Pulse oximetry is widely regarded as one of the greatest advances in clinical monitoring (Guiliano and Higgins, 2005) since the invention of the ECG

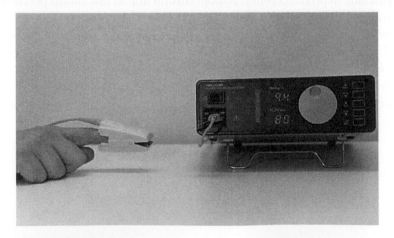

Figure 3.4 Pulse oximeter.

(Fox, 2002). It is a simple, non-invasive method of measuring arterial oxygen saturation (Higgins, 2005) expressed as SpO_2 (Welch, 2005). Pulse oximetry was developed in the 1980s; before this, oxygenation assessment was reliant on subjective and unreliable physical assessment of the skin for cyanosis (Guiliano and Higgins, 2005) which, when present, is an indicator of advanced hypoxaemia (Guiliano, 2006).

Pulse oximetry only measures the extent to which haemoglobin is saturated with oxygen and does not provide information on oxygen delivery to the tissues or ventilatory function (Higgins, 2005). Nevertheless, it is an invaluable monitoring tool in a variety of clinical settings, including in the dental practice when sedation is being administered to the patient.

Role of pulse oximetry

Hypoxaemia can occur in patients in the dental practice, e.g. while sedated or during a severe asthma attack. If unrecognised and untreated, it can lead to cellular death and organ dysfunction.

Cyanosis is a late sign of hypoxaemia and the oxygen saturation must decrease to 80–85% before any changes in skin colour become apparent (Guiliano and Higgins, 2005). In addition, manifestations of hypoxaemia including restlessness, confusion, agitation, cyanosis, combative behaviour and tachycardia may be missed or wrongly interpreted (Technology Subcommittee of the Working Group on Critical Care, 1992).

Pulse oximetry, the fifth vital sign (Welch, 2005) will immediately alert the dental practitioner to a fall in arterial oxygen saturations and the development of hypoxaemia, prior to visual recognition of cyanosis. In clinical practice an oxygen saturation of less than 90% is of concern.

The absence of cyanosis does not exclude severe hypoxaemia; it will not be present if the haemoglobin concentration is low or if there is poor perfusion of the capillaries

---

The mechanics of pulse oximetry

Pulse oximetry is a differential measurement based on the spectrophotometric absorption method using the Beer–Lambert Law for optical absorption (Welch, 2005).

The pulse oximeter probe consists of two light-emitting diodes (one red and one infrared) on one side of the probe. These transmit red and infrared light across the vascular bed, usually a fingertip or ear lobe, to a photodetector on the other side of the probe (Welch, 2005). The ratio of absorption is relative to the concentration of oxygenated haemoglobin to deoxygenated haemoglobin (Welch, 2005).

The more oxygenated the blood is, more red light passes through and less infrared light passes through (Guiliano, 2006). By calculating the ratios of red to infrared light change over time, oxygen saturation is calculated (Guiliano, 2006).

Uses of pulse oximetry in the dental practice

Pulse oximetry is indicated in any clinical situation where hypoxaemia may occur. In the dental practice it could be used in patients receiving sedation and acutely ill patients, e.g. severe asthma attack.

Advantages of pulse oximetry

Pulse oximetry is an inexpensive, non-invasive and portable method of continuous measurement of arterial oxygen saturation which facilitates the early detection of hypoxaemia. It also provides information about the heart rate (Welch, 2005).

Normal values for oxygen saturation

The normal range for oxygen saturation measurements is greater than 95% (Fox, 2002), though lower measurements may be 'normal' for some patients, e.g. those who have COPD (Fox, 2002).

Procedure for pulse oximetry

The following preliminary points should be observed (adapted from Jevon and Ewens, 2012).

- Ensure the probe is clean.
- Wash and dry hands.
- Explain the procedure to the patient.
- Select an appropriate site with an adequate pulsating vascular bed. Sites include finger (most popular) and ear lobe (less accurate); toes can be used instead of fingers, but this is generally not practical in the dental practice. In addition, poor perfusion is more common in the toes. If the finger is used, it is usual practice to remove any nail polish (Higgins, 2005) (obtain patient's consent first).
- Ensure that the trace is reliable and corresponds to pulse rate, i.e. oxygen saturation measurements are accurate.
- Ensure the alarms on the pulse oximeter are set within locally agreed limits and according to the patient's condition.
- Regularly monitor the patient's vital signs.
- Monitor the readings.

Causes of inaccuracy

Inaccurate readings can be caused by any of the factors listed below.

- *Carbon monoxide poisoning:* false high readings (Mathews, 2005).
- *Methemglobinaemia* (changes in the structure of iron in haemoglobin) and if present in high doses can give false high or low readings (Welch, 2005).
- *Poor vascular perfusion:* pulse oximeter requires pulsatile blood flow to evaluate oxygen saturation.
- *Venous pulsation:* e.g. tricuspid valve failure, securing the probe too tightly (Fox, 2002; Welch, 2005), heart failure, inflating blood pressure cuff distal to the probe, resulting in a false low reading.
- *Poor vascular perfusion:* e.g. in hypotension, anaphylactic shock or peripheral vascular disease, resulting in a false low reading.
- *Cardiac arrhythmias* such as atrial fibrillation can cause inadequate and irregular perfusion, resulting in a false low reading.
- *Factors that affect light absorption:* skin pigmentation, dried blood and dark nail polish (Welch, 2005).
- *Bright external light*, particularly fluorescent lighting (Fox, 2002; Gwinnutt, 2006) can give a false high reading.
- *Anaemia.*
- *Patient on supplementary oxygen* can mean that hypoxaemia will not be detected early.
- *Patient movement*, e.g. shivering; though modern pulse oximeters can minimise the interference from patient movement (Gwinnutt, 2006).

Limitations

Although pulse oximetry measures oxygen saturation and can detect hypoxaemia, it does not provide an indication of the adequacy of ventilation and carbon dioxide retention. Davidson and Hosie (1993) reported a case of a post-operative patient who had a normal oxygen saturation (95%), but had abnormally high carbon dioxide levels causing a life-threatening respiratory acidosis. Failure to detect hypoventilation in a patient is an example of a false sense of security generated by a single physiological variable being within safe limits. It is therefore paramount that, when using pulse oximetry, the dental practitioner is aware of its limitations and always monitors the patient's vital signs following the ABCDE approach.

Troubleshooting

It is important to ensure a reliable trace at all times. If it is difficult to secure an acceptable trace:

- warm and rub the skin to improve circulation;
- try a different probe site, e.g. ear lobe;
- try a different probe or a different pulse oximeter.

Complications

Pulse oximetry is very safe. Complications can occasionally occur, but generally only after prolonged use, which will not be the case in the dental practice.

PROCEDURE FOR ADMINISTERING OXYGEN TO THE ACUTELY ILL PATIENT

The non-rebreathing oxygen mask (Figure 3.1) enables the delivery of high concentrations of oxygen and is recommended for use in acutely ill patients (Resuscitation Council (UK), 2011). To ensure the mask is functioning correctly and is effectively used, it is important to follow the manufacturer's recommendations for simple basic checks prior to use (Intersurgical, 2003).

Description

The non-rebreathing mask (sometimes called a Hudson mask) with an oxygen reservoir bag can be used to deliver high concentrations of oxygen to a spontaneously breathing patient. A one-way valve diverts the oxygen flow into the reservoir bag during expiration; the contents of the reservoir bag together with the high flow oxygen, results in minimal entrainment of air and an inspired oxygen concentration of approximately 85% (Gwinnutt, 2006). The valve also prevents the patient's exhaled gases from entering the reservoir bag. The use of the oxygen reservoir bag helps to increase the inspired oxygen concentration by preventing oxygen loss during inspiration.

It is important to ensure that a sufficient oxygen flow rate is used to ensure that the oxygen reservoir bag does not collapse during inspiration (Resuscitation Council (UK), 2011). An oxygen flow rate of 12–15 l/min is recommended (Gwinnutt, 2006).

Procedure

- Ensure the patient is in an upright position to maximise breathing.
- If available in the dental practice, request that pulse oximetry is commenced.
- Explain the procedure to the patient.
- Attach the oxygen tubing to the oxygen source.
- Set the oxygen flow rate to 12–15 l/min (Gwinnutt, 2006).
- Occlude the valve between the mask and the oxygen reservoir bag (Figure 3.5) and check that the reservoir bag is filling up. Remove the finger.
- Squeeze the oxygen reservoir bag (Figure 3.6) to check the patency of the valve between the mask and the reservoir bag. If the valve is working

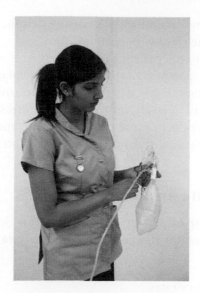

Figure 3.5 Checking the non-rebreathe mask; with oxygen 12–15 l attached, occlude the valve between the mask and the oxygen reservoir bag, checking that the reservoir bag fills up.

correctly it will be possible to empty the reservoir bag. If the reservoir bag does not empty, discard it and select another mask.

- Again occlude the valve between the mask and the oxygen reservoir bag, allowing the reservoir bag to fill up.
- Place the mask with a filled oxygen reservoir bag on the patient's face, ensuring a tight fit.

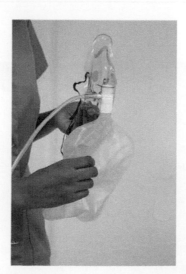

Figure 3.6 Checking the non-rebreathe mask: with oxygen 12–15 l attached, release the pressure on the valve and squeeze the oxygen reservoir bag – it should be empty.

- Adjust the oxygen flow rate sufficient to ensure that the reservoir bag deflates by approximately one-third with each breath.
- Provide reassurance to the patient.
- Closely monitor the patent's vital signs. In particular, assess the patient's response to the oxygen therapy, e.g. respiratory rate, mechanics of breathing, colour, oxygen saturation levels, level of consciousness.
- Discontinue or reduce the inspired oxygen concentration as appropriate following advice from the senior dental practitioner (Intersurgical, 2003).

Respiratory rate indicator

Some masks have a respiratory rate indicator (Figure 3.7) to help the healthcare practitioner to monitor the patient's respiratory rate. This indicator can be affected by:

- the patient's respiratory rate;
- the orientation of the indicator;
- the oxygen flow rate;
- the fit of the mask to the patient's face;
- the presence of moisture in the indicator tube – this can actually stop the indicator from working (Intersurgical, 2003).

> The respiratory rate indicator should only be used as a guide and should not replace close monitoring of the patient's breathing

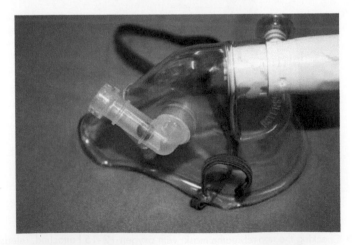

Figure 3.7 Respiratory rate indictor.

PROCEDURE FOR RECORDING BLOOD PRESSURE

Of all the measurements routinely undertaken in clinical practice, the recording of blood pressure is potentially the most unreliably and incorrectly performed measurement (British Hypertension Society, 2006a). It is essential that blood pressure recordings are accurate and reliable: good practice can significantly reduce measurement errors and help ensure that the blood pressure recording obtained is accurate and reliable.

Systolic and diastolic blood pressure

Systolic blood pressure is peak blood pressure in the artery following ventricular systole (contraction). *Diastolic blood pressure* is the level to which the arterial blood pressure falls during ventricular diastole (relaxation) (Talley and O'Connor, 2001).

Korotkoff sounds

Five different sound phases known as 'Korotkoff sounds' (Korotkoff, a Russian surgeon, first described the auscultation method of measuring blood pressure in 1905) can be heard as the blood pressure cuff is slowly released:

- Phase 1: a thud;
- Phase 2: a blowing or swishing noise;
- Phase 3: a softer thud than in sound 1;
- Phase 4: a disappearing blowing noise;
- Phase 5: silence (Talley and O'Connor, 2001; Dougherty and Lister, 2008).

Practically, the systolic reading is when the Korotkoff sounds are first heard and the diastolic reading is when the sounds disappear (British Hypertension Society, 2006a).

Which arm?

The blood pressure should initially be measured in both arms and the arm with the higher readings should be used for subsequent measurements (MHRA, 2005; NICE and British Hypertension Society, 2006). Although a difference in blood pressure measurements between the arms can be expected in 20% of patients, if this difference is >20 mm Hg for systolic or >10 mm Hg for diastolic on three consecutive readings, further investigation will probably be indicated (MHRA, 2005; NICE and British Hypertension Society, 2006).

Procedure for manual measurement of a blood pressure

The traditional manual blood pressure device (Figure 3.8) using auscultation is still very popular, and when used correctly, a reliable method of recording blood pressure. The following procedure for its use is recommended.

- Ideally ensure that the patient has been resting for at least 5 minutes and is comfortably relaxed.
- Check the equipment, ensuring it is in good working order.
- Explain the procedure to the patient and obtain his consent.
- Ask the patient to remove any tight clothing from around his arm.
- Ensure the patient's arm is supported at the level of the heart. If the arm is unsupported, the blood pressure is likely to be erroneously increased due to muscle contraction in the arm. If the arm is higher than the level of the heart, this can lead to an underestimation of the diastolic pressure by as much as 10 mm Hg (MHRA, 2005).
- Select an appropriately sized cuff: the bladder of the cuff should encircle at least 80% of the arm but no more than 100%.
- Place the cuff snugly onto the patient's arm, with the centre of the bladder over the brachial artery – most cuffs have a 'brachial artery indicator', an arrow which will be aligned with the brachial artery.
- Position the manometer near to the patient. It should be vertical and at the practitioner's eye level.
- Ask the patient to refrain from talking as this can result in an inaccurate higher blood pressure.

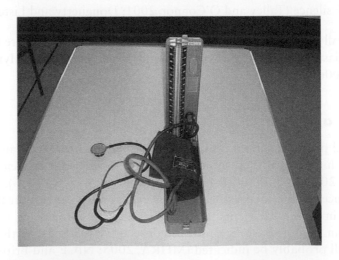

Figure 3.8 Mercury sphygmomanometer.

- Estimate the systolic pressure: palpate the brachial artery, inflate the cuff and note the reading when the brachial pulse disappears. Then deflate the cuff.
- Inflate the cuff to 30 mm Hg above the estimated systolic level, which was required to occlude the brachial pulse. Approximately 5% of the population has an auscultatory gap; this is when the Korotkoff sounds disappear just below the systolic pressure and reappear above the diastolic pressure (Talley and O'Connor, 2001). Estimating the systolic pressure will help ensure that the cuff is sufficiently inflated to record an accurate systolic pressure.
- Palpate the brachial artery.
- Place the diaphragm of the stethoscope gently over the brachial artery. Avoid applying excessive pressure on the diaphragm and do not tuck the diaphragm under the edge of the cuff because either of these actions could partially occlude the brachial artery, delaying the occurrence of the Korotkoff sounds (Figure 3.9).
- Open the valve and slowly deflate the cuff at a rate of 2–3 mm/s, recording when the Korotkoff sounds first appear (systolic) and disappear (diastolic).
- Document the systolic and diastolic blood pressure readings on the patient's observation chart following local protocols. Compare with previous readings and inform the nurse in charge/medical team as appropriate.

Source: British Hypertension Society (2006a, 2006b), NICE and British Hypertension Society (2006)

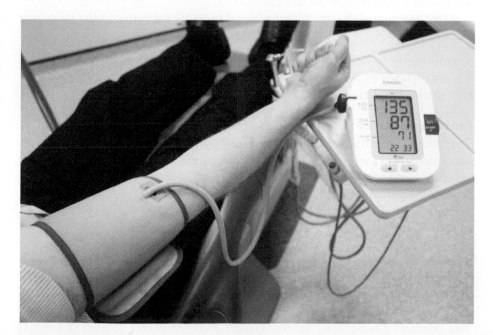

Figure 3.9 Manual blood pressure measurement.

Errors in blood pressure measurement

Errors in blood pressure measurement can occur for several reasons (British Hypertension Society, 2006a) including:

- Defective equipment, e.g. leaking tubing or a faulty valve;
- Failure to ensure the mercury column reads 0 mm Hg at rest;
- Too rapid deflation of the cuff;
- Use of incorrectly sized cuff: if it is too small the blood pressure will be over-estimated and if it is too big the blood pressure will be underestimated;
- Cuff not at the same level as the heart;
- Failure to observe the mercury level properly – the top of the mercury column should be at eye level;
- Poor technique (e.g. failing to note when the sounds disappear);
- Digit preference, rounding the reading up to the nearest 5 or 10 mm Hg;
- Observer bias, e.g. expecting a young patient's blood pressure to be normal.

Automated blood pressure devices

When automated blood pressure devices were first manufactured, their accuracy and reliability was questioned (Beevers *et al.*, 2001). However, improved technology has led to the development of more accurate and reliable devices (Beevers *et al.*, 2001), some of which have been tested and approved for use by the British Hypertension Society (2006a).

Most automated devices measure blood pressure using one of the following techniques:

- oscillometry to detect arterial blood flow (most commonly used device);
- a microphone to detect the Korotkoff sounds;
- ultrasound to detect arterial blood flow (British Hypertension Society, 2006a).

Procedure for automated measurement of blood pressure

The principles for the accurate measurement of blood pressure using an automated electronic device will be similar to the manual recording of blood pressure using a sphygmomanometer in respect of preparing the patient, positioning the patient and choice and placement of cuff. However, when using an automated electronic device, it is important to be familiar with its working and to follow the manufacturer's recommendations when using it.

MEDICAL EMERGENCIES IN THE DENTAL PRACTICE POSTER

The *Medical Emergencies in the Dental Practice* poster (Figure 3.10) has been designed by Walsall healthcare NHS Trust to help dental practitioners

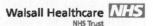

Figure 3.10 'Medical Emergencies in the Dental Practice' poster. *Source*: Walsall Healthcare NHS Trust. Reproduced with permission.

recognize and effectively treat and manage medical emergencies in the dental practice. Each emergency is listed alphabetically, together with the signs and symptoms for each one. The treatment for each emergency is listed in a bullet point approach format, facilitating a tick-box exercise helping to ensure that the priorities of treatment are performed and nothing important is overlooked. Drug doses, including paediatric doses where appropriate, are also included. The poster can be downloaded free of charge from www.walsallhealthcare. nhs.uk

CONCLUSION

This chapter has provided an overview to the principles of recognition of the sick patient. The clinical signs of acute illness have been listed and the ABCDE approach has been discussed and described.

REFERENCES

Beevers G, Marshall T, Rouse A (2001) Blood pressure measurement part 1: sphygmomanometry: factors common to all techniques. *British Medical Journal*; 322:981–985.

British Hypertension Society (2006a) *Blood Pressure Measurement with Mercury Blood Pressure Monitors,* www.bhsoc.org (accessed 20 April 2013).

British Hypertension Society (2006b) *Let's Do It Well,* http://www.bhsoc.org/pdfs/hit.pdf (accessed 20 April 2013).

British Thoracic Society (2008) *2008 British Guideline on the Management of Asthma.* British Thoracic Society, London.

Buist M, Jarmolowski E, Burton P *et al.* (1999) Recognising clinical instability in hospital patients before cardiac arrest or unplanned admission to intensive care. *Medical Journal of Australia*; 171:22–25.

Davidson J, Hosie H (1993) Limitations of pulse oximetry: respiratory insufficiency – a failure of detection. *British Medical Journal*; 307:372–373.

Dougherty L, Lister S (2008) *The Royal Marsden Hospital Manual of Clinical Nursing Procedures*, 7th edn. Wiley-Blackwell Publishing, Oxford.

Ford M, Hennessey I, Japp A (2005) *Introduction to Clinical Examination*. Elsevier, Oxford.

Fox N (2002) Pulse oximetry. *Nursing Times*; 98(40):65–67.

Goldhill DR, Worthington L, Mulcahy A *et al.* (1999) The patient-at-risk team: identifying and managing seriously ill patients. *Anaesthesia*; 54:853–860.

Goldhill D, McNarry A (2004) Physiological abnormalities in early warning scores are related to mortality in adult inpatients. *British Journal of Anaesthesia*; 92(6):882–884.

Greenwood M (2009) Medical Emergencies in Dental Practice: 1. The Drug Box, Equipment and General Approach *Dental Update*; 36: 202–211

Guiliano K, Higgins T (2005) New-generation pulse oximetry in the care of critically ill patients. *American Journal of Critical Care*; 14:26–37.

Guiliano K (2006) Knowledge of pulse oximetry among critical care nurses. *Dimensions of Critical Care Nursing*; 25(1):44–49.

Gwinnutt C (2006) *Clinical Anaesthesia*, 2nd edn. Wiley-Blackwell Publishing, Oxford.

Higgins D (2005) Oxygen therapy. *Nursing Times*; 101(4):30–31.

Intersurgical (2003) *Non-rebreathing mask product literature*. Intersurgical, Wokingham.

Jevon P, Ewens B (2012) *Monitoring the Critically ill Patient 3rd Ed* Wiley Oxford

Mathews P (2005) The latest in respiratory care. *Nursing Management supplement: critical care choices*; 18:20–21.

MHRA (2005) *Report of the Independent Advisory Group on Blood Pressure Monitoring in Clinical Practice*. Medicine and Healthcare products Regulatory Agency, London.

NICE & the British Hypertension Society (2006) *NICE/BHS Hypertension Guideline Review*, 28 June 2006 http://www.bhsoc.org/NICE_BHS_Guidelines.stm (accessed 20 April 2013).

Nolan J, Deakin C, Soar J et al. (2005) European Resuscitation Council Guidelines for Resuscitation 2005. Section 4. Adult advanced life support. *Resuscitation*; 67 (Suppl 1): S39–S86.

Resuscitation Council (UK) (2012) *Medical Emergencies and Resuscitation Standards for Clinical Practice and Training for Dental Practitioners and Dental Care Professionals in General Dental Practice*. Resuscitation Council (UK), London.

Resuscitation Council (UK) (2011) *Advanced Life Support*, 6th edn. Resuscitation Council (UK), London.

Talley N, O'Connor S (2001) *Clinical Examination: A Systematic Guide to Physical Diagnosis*. Blackwell Science, Oxford.

Technology Subcommittee of the Working Group on Critical Care (1992) Non-invasive gas monitoring: a review for use in the adult critical care unit. *Canadian Medical Association Journal*; 146:703–712.

Welch J (2005) Pulse oximeters. *Biomedical Instrumentation and Technology*; 39(2):125–130.

RECOGNITION AND TREATMENT OF THE ACUTELY ILL PATIENT

Chapter 4

Respiratory disorders

INTRODUCTION

In the United Kingdom, respiratory disorders account for 20% of all deaths; in 2004, 117,000 deaths were caused by respiratory disease compared to 106,000 deaths from ischaemic heart disease (British Thoracic Society, 2006). Mortality rates from respiratory disease have remained static over the last 20 years (British Thoracic Society, 2006). Social class inequality is estimated to be associated with 44% of all deaths from respiratory disease (British Thoracic Society, 2006).

The common occurrence of respiratory disease in the United Kingdom guarantees that it will be encountered in the dental practice. If serious, it can be life threatening. It is essential to assess the patient following the ABCDE approach described in Chapter 3.

The aim of this chapter is to understand the management of respiratory disorders.

LEARNING OUTCOMES

At the end of the chapter the reader will be able to:

- Discuss the management of an acute asthma attack
- Discuss the management of hyperventilation
- Discuss the management of exacerbation of chronic obstructive pulmonary disease (COPD)
- Describe the procedure for using an inhaler device
- Describe the procedure for using a spacer device

MANAGEMENT OF ACUTE ASTHMA ATTACK

There is no standard definition of asthma, though central to all definitions is the presence of key characteristics of the disease, i.e. one or more of wheeze, breathlessness, chest tightness and cough (British Thoracic Society, 2008).

There is considerable variation between patients in respect of the severity of episodes they experience and the overall course of the disease; for some patients their illness is well controlled and they are asymptomatic between acute attacks while for others the illness can progress to a state of irreversible airway obstruction (Bourke, 2003).

Incidence

It is estimated that in the United Kingdom 5.4 million people have asthma, of whom 1.1 million are children and 4.3 million are adults (Asthma UK, 2013). Although the number of children with asthma has fallen since a peak in the 1990s, the number of adults with asthma is on the increase.

In the United Kingdom, there are approximately 80,000 hospital admissions for asthma each year and 1400 deaths were attributed to asthma (Asthma UK, 2013). Although the incidence of acute asthma episodes in primary care is on the decline (Sunderland and Fleming, 2004), it is nevertheless important to be vigilant. Asthma-related emergencies account for 5% of all medical emergencies encountered in the dental practice (Müller *et al.*, 2008).

Pathogenesis

Asthma is characterised by episodes of reversible airway obstruction where hypersensitivity to certain triggers sets off an inflammatory response during which mucus is released and the muscles of the bronchi constrict (Ward *et al*, 2010). The inflammatory process involves infiltration of the airway walls by various immune cells, oedema, hypertrophy of mucus glands and damage to the airway epithelial wall (Deacon, 2008). This airway remodelling from persistent inflammation can lead to permanent fibrotic damage.

Causes

Causes of an asthma attack include:

• smoking;
• dust;
• animals;

- stress;
- chest infection.

Source: Ward *et al.* (2010), Asthma UK (2013)

In the dental practice, stress can trigger an acute asthma attack (Müller *et al.*, 2008).

Signs and symptoms

Signs and symptoms of asthma include:

- wheeze;
- shortness of breath;
- chest tightness;
- cough.

Source: British Thoracic Society (2008)

The hallmark of asthma is that these symptoms tend to be:

- variable;
- intermittent;
- worse at night;
- provoked by triggers including stress.

Source: Jevon (2006)

The speed of onset of an acute asthma attack can vary; although there is normally a history of deterioration over a period of days or weeks, an attack can sometimes occur suddenly with rapid deterioration (Rees and Kanabar, 2007).

The severity of acute asthma can range from moderate to life threatening (Figure 4.1) (British Thoracic Society, 2008).

Patients with severe or life-threatening asthma may not be distressed; they could be quiet and drowsy (pre-cardiopulmonary arrest situation)

Treatment

The British Thoracic Society has issued guidelines on the management of acute asthma (Figure 4.1).

- Assess the patient following the ABCDE approach described in Chapter 3.
- Sit the patient up (Wyatt *et al.*, 2012).

Management of acute severe asthma in adults in general practice

Many deaths from asthma are preventable. Delay can be fatal. Factors leading to poor outcome include:

- Clinical staff. Failing to assess severity by objective measurement
- Patients or relatives failing to appreciate severity
- Under-use of corticosteroids

Regard each emergency asthma consultation as for acute severe asthma until shown otherwise.

Assess and record:

- Peak expiratory flow (PEF)
- Symptoms and response to self treatment
- Heart and respiratory rates
- Oxygen saturation (by pulse oximetry)

Caution: Patients with severe or life threatening attacks may not be distressed and may not have all the abnormalities listed below. The presence of any should alert the doctor.

Moderate asthma	Acute severe asthma	Life threatening asthma
INITIAL ASSESSMENT		
PEF > 50-75% best or predicted	PEF 33-50% best or predicted	PEF < 33% best or predicted
FURTHER ASSESSMENT		
■ SpO$_2$ ≥ 92% ■ Speech normal ■ Respiration <25 breaths/min ■ Pulse <110 beats/min	■ SpO$_2$ ≥ 92% ■ Can't complete sentences ■ Respiration ≥25 breaths/min ■ Pulse ≥110 beats/min	■ SpO$_2$ <92% ■ Silent chest, cyanosis or poor respiratory effort ■ Arrhythmia or hypotension ■ Exhaustion, altered consciousness
MANAGEMENT		
Treat at home or in surgery and ASSESS RESPONSE TO TREATMENT	Consider admission	Arrange immediate ADMISSION
TREATMENT		
■ β$_2$ bronchodilator: - - Via spacer (give 4 puffs initially and give a further 2 puffs every 2 minutes according to response up to maximum of 10 puffs) If PEF > 50-75% predicted/best: ■ nebuliser (preferably oxygen driven) (salbutamol 5 mg or terbutaline 10 mg) ■ Give prednisolone 40-50 mg ■ Continue or step up usual treatment If good response to first treatment *(symptoms improved, respiration and pulse settling and PEF >50%)* continue or step up usual treatment and continue prednisolone	■ Oxygen to maintain SpO$_2$ 94-98% if available ■ β$_2$ bronchodilator: - nebuliser (preferably oxygen driven) (salbutamol 5 mg or terbutaline 10 mg) - Or via spacer (give 4 puffs initially and give a further 2 puffs every 2 minutes according to response up to maximum of 10 puffs) ■ Prednisolone 40-50 mg or IV hydrocortisone 100 mg ■ **If no response in acute severe asthma: ADMIT**	■ Oxygen to maintain SpO$_2$ 94-98% ■ β$_2$ bronchodilator and ipratropium: - nebuliser (preferably oxygen driven) (salbutamol 5 mg or terbutaline 10 mg) and (ipratropium 0.5mg) - Or via spacer (give 4 puffs initially and give a further 2 puffs every 2 minutes according to response up to maximum of 10 puffs) ■ Prednisolone 40-50 mg or IV hydrocortisone 100 mg immediately
Admit to hospital if any: ■ life threatening features ■ features of acute severe asthma present after initial treatment ■ previous near-fatal asthma Lower threshold for admission if afternoon or evening attack, recent nocturnal symptoms or hospital admission, previous severe attacks, patient unable to assess own condition, or concern over social circumstances.	**If admitting the patient to hospital:** ■ Stay with patient until ambulance arrives ■ Send written asssessment and referral details to hospital ■ β$_2$ bronchodilator via oxygen-driven nebuliser in ambulance	**Follow up after treatment or discharge from hospital:** ■ **GP review within 48 hours** ■ Monitor symptoms and PEF ■ Check inhaler technique ■ Written asthma action plan ■ Modify treatment according to guidelines for chronic persistent asthma ■ Address potentially preventable contributors to admission

Figure 4.1 British Thoracic Society (2008) guidelines on the management of acute asthma (Reproduced with kind permission).

- If available, consult the patient's individual action plan in the event of an asthma attack (British Thoracic Society, 2008).
- Encourage the patient to take two puffs of a short-acting beta-2 adrenoceptor stimulant inhaler, e.g. salbutamol (100 µg/puff) (Figure 4.2) (British Medical Association and Royal Pharmaceutical Society, 2013). Hopefully the patient will be using his own inhaler and should therefore be familiar with its use and will be administering what his own general practitioner has prescribed. However, if he does not have this with him, use the inhaler stored in the emergency drugs box in the dental practice. (A suggested procedure for using an inhaler is described later.)
- If the patient does not rapidly respond, administer further puffs (British Medical Association and Royal Pharmaceutical Society, 2013).
- If the patient is unable to take his inhaler effectively, administer further puffs through a spacer device (Figure 4.3) (see Procedure for using a spacer device); if one is not available, a plastic or paper cup with a hole in the bottom for the inhaler mouthpiece will suffice (Figure 4.4) (British Medical Association and Royal Pharmaceutical Society, 2013).
- If the patient does not respond satisfactorily or if deterioration occurs, call 999 for an ambulance; while awaiting transfer to hospital, administer oxygen and also salbutamol 2.5–5 mg via a nebuliser (if this is not available, administer 4–10 puffs of salbutamol 100 µg/puff inhaler preferably via a large volume spacer device, repeating every 20 minutes if necessary (British Medical Association and Royal Pharmaceutical Society, 2013).

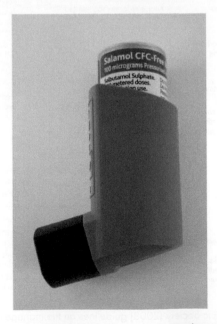

Figure 4.2 Example of a short-acting beta-2 adrenoceptor stimulant inhaler.

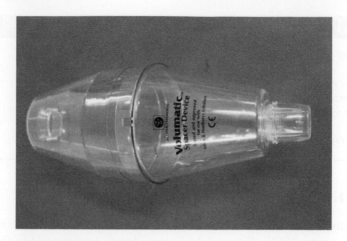

Figure 4.3 Spacer device.

- Monitor the patient following the ABCDE approach, with particular attention to respiratory rate, heart rate and level of consciousness (British Thoracic Society, 2008; Wyatt *et al.*, 2012) (Boxes 4.1 and 4.2).
- Reassure the patient; an acute asthma attack is frightening and the need to be admitted to hospital can increase anxiety and exacerbate symptoms (Rees and Kanabar, 2007).

Source: Jevon (2006), British Medical Association and Royal Pharmaceutical Society (2013), British Thoracic Society (2008)

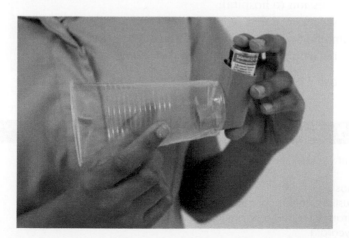

Figure 4.4 Spacer device not available: a plastic or paper cup with a hole in the bottom for the inhaler mouthpiece will suffice (British Medical Association and Pharmaceutical Society of Great Britain, 2013).

RESPIRATORY DISORDERS

RESPIRATORY DISORDERS

Box 4.1   Signs of acute severe asthma

A patient with asthma with any one of the following:

- Inability to complete sentences in one breath
- Respiratory rate of 25 or more per minute
- Heart rate of 110 or more per minute

Source: Wyatt *et al.* (2012).

Indications for hospital admission

Asthma has been classified into moderate, severe and life threatening (British Thoracic Society, 2008) (Figure 4.1). For moderate, severe and life-threatening asthma, the following is recommended:

- *Moderate asthma:* treat at home or in the surgery and assess response to treatment;
- *Severe asthma:* immediate transfer to hospital should be arranged if the casualty is not responding to treatment;
- *Life-threatening asthma:* immediate transfer to hospital should be arranged.

Source: Resuscitation Council (UK) (2012), British Thoracic Society (2008)

Factors lowering the threshold for hospital admission include:

- Afternoon or evening episode;
- Recent nocturnal symptoms;
- Recent admission to hospital;
- Previous severe episodes;
- Patient unable to assess own condition;
- Concern regarding the patient's social circumstances.

Source: British Thoracic Society (2008), Rees and Kanabar (2007)

Box 4.2   Signs of life-threatening asthma

A patient with asthma with any one of the following:

- Cyanosis
- Exhaustion, confusion, coma
- Respiratory effort < 8 per minute
- Bradycardia

Source: British Thoracic Society (2008), Wyatt *et al.* (2012).

Factors that contribute to a poor outcome

Factors that contribute to a poor outcome include:

• Healthcare practitioners failing to assess severity by objective measurement;
• Patients or relatives failing to recognise the severity of an attack;
• Underuse of corticosteroids.

Source: British Thoracic Society (2008)

Most deaths caused by asthma are preventable, but delay in referring the patient to hospital could be fatal (British Thoracic Society, 2008). Mortality is usually associated with failure to appreciate the severity of the exacerbation, leading to inadequate emergency treatment and delay in referring to hospital (British Thoracic Society, 2008).

MANAGEMENT OF HYPERVENTILATION

Hyperventilation can be defined as a fast respiratory rate resulting in an increased loss of carbon dioxide (Soanes and Stevenson, 2006). It is usually anxiety induced and may accompany a panic attack (Jevon, 2006). It can occur in a susceptible person who has recently experienced emotional or psychological trauma (St John Ambulance *et al.*, 2011) and is not uncommon in the dental practice. It may be associated with attention-seeking behaviour.

Hyperventilation can lead to hypocapnia (low carbon dioxide levels in the blood) causing tingling in the extremities and the mouth, dizziness, trembling and cramps. Sometimes it can be mistaken for anaphylaxis (Resuscitation

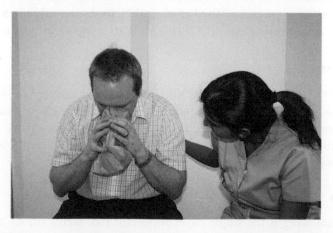

Figure 4.5 Management of hyperventilation: reassurance.

RESPIRATORY DISORDERS

Council (UK), 2012), particularly if the patient starts to hyperventilate follow-ing the administration of a local anaesthetic. It is therefore always important to carefully assess the patient following the ABCDE approach so that serious illness can be excluded (Wyatt *et al.*, 2012).

Treatment

- Reassure the patient; it may be necessary to be firm;
- If possible remove the cause of the distress or anxiety;
- If possible take the patient somewhere private where he can regain control of his breathing again;
- Try simple breathing exercises, e.g. breathe in through nose counting up to eight, breathe out through mouth counting up to eight and then hold breath-ing counting up to four and repeat.

Source: St John Ambulance *et al.* (2011), Wyatt *et al.* (2012)

NB: Although, it is no longer recommended to advise the patient to rebreathe his own exhaled air from a paper bag because this may cause a more serious illness (St John Ambulance *et al.*, 2011), this technique is still sometimes used (caution) (Figure 4.5).

MANAGEMENT OF EXACERBATION OF CHRONIC OBSTRUCTIVE PULMONARY DISEASE

COPD describes a spectrum of disease processes characterised by a chronic and progressive reduction in airflow (Deacon, 2008). COPD encompasses chronic bronchitis and emphysema that often present together but reflect dif-ferent underlying processes (Ward *et al.*, 2010). In the dental practice a patient could have an exacerbation of COPD leading to acute breathlessness.

Incidence

Over 600,000 people in the United Kingdom have been diagnosed with COPD (a prevalence of 1%) (Calverly and Bellamy, 2000). Socioeconomic factors play a strong role in COPD: men aged 20–64 years who work in manual unskilled jobs are 14 times more likely to die from COPD than those in profes-sional jobs (British Thoracic Society, 2006).

Causes

Cigarette smoking is the single most important risk factor for COPD (British Thoracic Society, 2008).

Clinical features

There is great variability in the symptoms experienced by patients with different severities of airflow obstruction and in the rate of disease progression (Deacon, 2008). However, the key clinical features are cough, wheeze and breathlessness (Halpin, 2003). A productive cough is common.

Treatment

If a patient with COPD presents with acute shortness of breath in the dental practice:

- Assess the patient following the ABCDE approach described in Chapter 3.
- Ensure the patient has a clear airway.
- Sit the patient in an upright position and administer oxygen. All critically ill patients should receive oxygen, even COPD patients in whom high concentrations of oxygen may depress respiratory function; these patients will sustain organ damage or cardiac arrest if their blood oxygen tensions are allowed to fall; the aim in this group of patients is to achieve a lower than normal PaO_2 (e.g. 8 kPa) or oxygen concentration (e.g. 90–92%) (Resuscitation Council (UK), 2012).
- If available, commence pulse oximetry.
- If indicated, encourage the patient to take two puffs of a short-acting beta-2 adrenoceptor stimulant inhaler, e.g. salbutamol (100 µg/puff) (Figure 4.2) (National Institute for Clinical Excellence, 2004).
- Monitor the patient's level of consciousness using the AVPU scale (Chapter 3); if the patient's level of consciousness starts to deteriorate, e.g. he becomes drowsy, this is an adverse sign because it may indicate that he is becoming hypoxic and/or hypercapnic (rising levels of carbon dioxide).
- Consider the need to dial 999 for an ambulance.

PROCEDURE FOR USING AN INHALER

An inhaler is a device for the administration of an inhalation (McFerran and Martin, 2003). Various inhalers and formulations have been developed to help ensure the efficient delivery of drugs, simply and with minimal side effects (Rees and Kanabar, 2007). Various different devices are available, the most common being the pressurized metered dose inhaler (pMDI) (Figure 4.2). This type is available in most emergency drug boxes in dental practices. For the purpose of this book, the term inhaler will suffice.

RESPIRATORY DISORDERS

Types of inhaler

Pressurized metered dose inhalers (pMDIs) (Figure 4.2) are the commonest type of inhaler used. They are small, convenient, easy to carry and deliver a wide range of medications (Newell and Hume, 2006). However, the correct technique for using a pMDI can be difficult to master because it requires co-ordinating actuation and inhalation efficiently, and inhaling at the correct inspiratory flow rate (Pearce, 2000).

Some patients, particularly the elderly and small children, find it difficult to use a pMDI (British Medical Association and Royal Pharmaceutical Society, 2013). Patients with arthritis may also struggle to use them correctly (Rees and Kanabar, 2007). The use of the pMDI should therefore be reserved for patients who can consistently demonstrate that they can use them correctly (Pearce, 2000). Except for the Seretide Evohaler, the pMDI does not have a dose counter and some users require to estimate when it is nearly empty (Newell and Hume, 2006).

Breath-actuated inhalers (*Autohaler* and *Easi-Breathe*) are also small and easy to carry. As inhalation on the mouthpiece triggers the dose of medication to be released, they do not require the user to co-ordinate actuation and inhalation, which is an obvious advantage over pMDIs (Newell and Hume, 2006).

Dry powder inhalers (e.g. Accuhaler, Diskhaler) deliver the inhaled medication in the form of a dry powder. They are activated by the patient's inspiratory effort, thus automatically actuating the device (Newell and Hume, 2006). Although they are popular and generally easy to use, some devices require a fairly high respiratory flow rate in order to be activated (Newell and Hume, 2006).

Drugs administered using an inhaler

Drugs that can be administered using an inhaler include (Currie and Douglas, 2007):

- *Short-acting beta-2 agonists, e.g. salbutamol:* act on beta-2 adrenoreceptors in bronchial smooth muscle causing bronchodilation that improves lung function and reduces breathlessness; effective for up to 6 hours. The Resuscitation Council (UK) recommends that a salbutamol inhaler should be kept in the dental practice (Resuscitation Council (UK), 2012).
- *Short-acting anticholinergics, e.g. ipratropium:* inhibit the action of acetylcholine resulting in relaxation of smooth muscle and bronchodilation that improves lung function and reduces breathlessness; effective for up to 6 hours.
- *Long-acting beta-2 agonists, e.g. salmeterol:* effective for up to 12 hours.
- *Long-acting anticholinergics, e.g. tiotropium:* effective for up to 24 hours.

RESPIRATORY DISORDERS

Drug delivery using an inhaler

An inhaler is designed to deliver the correct dose of an inhalation to an appropriate part of the airway. Even when an inhaler is used properly, only 10% of the drug reaches the airways below the larynx; 50% is deposited in the mouth, with close to 90% eventually being swallowed (Currie and Douglas, 2007; Rees and Kanabar, 2007).

Procedure

The procedure for the use of an inhaler, the commonest inhaler and the one usually available in the dental practice's emergency drug box, will now be described (Pearce, 2000; Jevon and Humphrey, 2007a; Currie and Douglas, 2007).

- Explain the procedure to the patient.
- Ask the patient to remove the mouthpiece cover from the inhaler (Figure 4.6).
- Ask the patient to shake the metered-dose inhaler and then breathe out slowly.
- Advise the patient to place the mouthpiece into his mouth and to close his lips and teeth around it.
- At the start of inspiration, ask the patient to press the canister down while he continues to inhale slowly and deeply (Figure 4.7).
- Advise the patient to remove the mouthpiece from his mouth and to then close his lips.

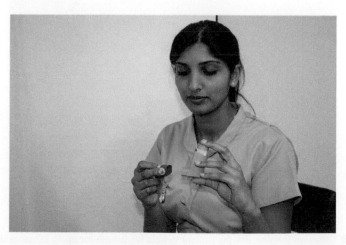

Figure 4.6 Using an inhaler: remove the mouthpiece cover from the inhaler.

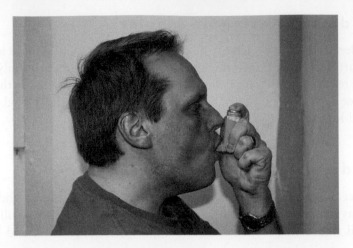

Figure 4.7 Using an inhaler: at the start of inspiration, ask the patient to press the canister down while he continues to inhale slowly and deeply.

- Ask the patient to hold his breath for up to 10 seconds (or as long as it is comfortable to do so) and then to breathe out normally (Figure 4.8).
- If a second dose is required, wait 30 seconds and repeat the above steps before replacing the cover.
- Document that the inhaler has been administered.
- The use of the inhaler with a spacer device is recommended for some patients.

Source: Asthma UK (2013)

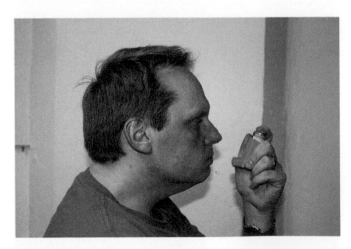

Figure 4.8 Using an inhaler: ask the patient to hold his breath for up to 10 seconds and then to breathe out normally.

Procedures for using other inhalers

It is not possible to describe the use of all the different inhalers currently available. It is important to refer to the manufacturers' recommendations for the correct use of their inhalers.

Teaching and monitoring the patient

The patient should be carefully instructed on how to use his inhaler and it is important to ensure that he continues to use it correctly because inadequate inhalation technique may be mistaken for a lack of response to the prescribed drug (British Medical Association and Royal Pharmaceutical Society, 2013). Asthma UK's website contains detailed advice on how to correctly use inhalers which the patient may find helpful: www.asthma.org.uk

PROCEDURE FOR USING A SPACER DEVICE

A spacer device is a large plastic or metal container, with a mouthpiece at one end and a hole for the aerosol inhaler at the other (Asthma UK, 2013). It is basically a chamber that acts as a reservoir for the aerosol cloud, removing the need for co-ordinating actuation of a pMDI and inhalation (Pearce, 2000).

A spacer device will only work with an aerosol inhaler (Asthma UK, 2013). When used correctly, an inhaler with a spacer device attached is at least as effective as any other device for delivering inhaled drugs (Currie and Douglas, 2007).

Types of spacer device

Several spacer devices are currently available; the larger ones with a one-way valve, e.g. Nebuhaler Volumatic, are the most effective (British Medical Association and Royal Pharmaceutical Society, 2013).

Advantages of using a spacer device

Advantages of using a spacer device include:

- making aerosol inhalers easier to use: removes the need for co-ordination between actuation of an inhaler and inhalation;
- reducing the velocity of the aerosol and subsequent impaction on the patient's oropharynx;
- allowing more time for the propellant to evaporate, thus enabling a larger proportion of the drug particles to be inhaled and deposited in the lungs;

RESPIRATORY DISORDERS

RESPIRATORY DISORDERS

- reducing the risk of side effects from the higher doses of preventer medicines by reducing the amount of medicine that is swallowed and absorbed into the body.

Source: British Medical Association and Royal Pharmaceutical Society (2013), Asthma UK (2013)

Indications

Indications for using a spacer device include:

- patients with poor inhaler technique;
- children and infants;
- patients requiring high doses of medications.

Principles of using a spacer

- The spacer should be compatible with the inhaler that is being used.
- The drug should be administered by repeated single actuations of the metered dose inhaler into the spacer, each followed by an inhalation.
- There should be minimal delay between inhaler actuation and inhalation.
- Tidal breathing is just as effective as single breaths (British Thoracic Society, 2008).

Procedure

- Ensure the space device is compatible to the inhaler being used.
- If necessary, assemble the spacer device (some devices come in two halves) (Figure 4.9).

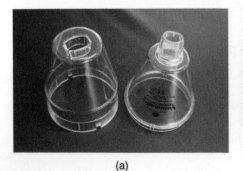
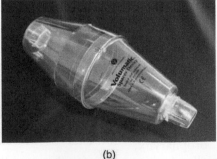

(a)   (b)

Figure 4.9 (a), (b) Using a spacer device: assemble if necessary.

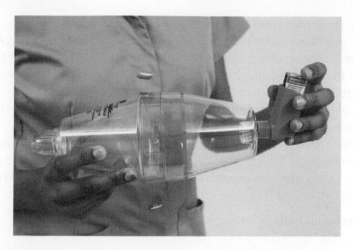

Figure 4.10 Using a spacer device: remove the cap from the mouthpiece on the inhaler and fit the latter to the spacer device.

- Shake the inhaler.
- Remove the cap from the mouthpiece on the MDI and fit the MDI to the spacer device (Figure 4.10).
- Close lips and teeth around mouthpiece.
- Actuate the MDI.
- Inhale deeply and slowly; ask the patient to hold his breath for 10 seconds (or as long as it is comfortable) – inhalation should be as soon as possible following actuation, definitely within 30 seconds (Rees and Kanabar, 2007) (Figure 4.11).

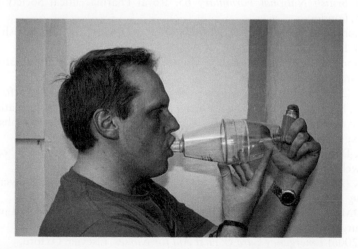

Figure 4.11 Using a spacer device: ask the patient to inhale deeply and slowly, then hold his breath for 10 seconds (or as long as it is comfortable).

- Remove the device from the mouth and close lips.
- Breathe out slowly (Asthma UK, 2013). It is recommended to take at least two deeply held breaths for each puff of the inhaler (Asthma UK, 2013). Some patients may find it difficult to take deep breaths – normal tidal breathing is considered just as effective (Asthma UK, 2013).
- If a second dose is required, wait 30 seconds before repeating the above procedure (Asthma UK, 2013).
- In infants and children under 2 years of age, attach a mask to the spacer device to facilitate its effective use; also hold the spacer at an angle of 45° to keep the valve open – the medication can then be inhaled during normal tidal breathing (Rees and Kanabar, 2007).

Source: Jevon and Humphrey (2007b)

CONCLUSION

Respiratory disorders can occur in the dental practice. In this chapter the management of an acute asthma attack, hyperventilation and exacerbation of COPD have been discussed. In addition, the procedures for using an inhaler device and a spacer device have been described.

REFERENCES

Asthma UK (2013) www.asthma.org.uk (accessed 14 March 2013).
British Medical Association & the Royal Pharmaceutical Society of Great Britain (2013) *British National Formulary 65.* Royal Pharmaceutical Society of Great Britain, London
British Thoracic Society (2006) *The Burden of Lung Disease,* 2nd edn. British Thoracic Society, London.
British Thoracic Society (2008) *British Guideline on the Management of Asthma.* British Thoracic Society, London.
Bourke SJ (2003) *Respiratory Medicine,* 6th edn. Blackwell Publishing, Oxford.
Calverly P, Bellamy D (2000) The challenge of providing better care for patients with chronic obstructive pulmonary disease: the poor relation of airways obstruction? *Thorax*; 55(1):78–82.
Currie G, Douglas J (2007) Oxygen and inhalers. In: Currie G (ed) *ABC of COPD,* Blackwell Publishing, Oxford.
Deacon K (2008) Respiratory emergencies. In: Jevon P, Humphreys M, Ewens B (eds) *Nursing Medical Emergency Patients.* Wiley-Blackwell, Oxford.
Halpin DMG (2003) *Your Questions Answered – COPD.* Churchill Livingstone, Edinburgh.
Jevon P (2006) *Emergency Care & First Aid for Nurses.* Elsevier, Oxford.
Jevon P, Humphrey N (2007a) Respiratory procedures part 5: use of an inhaler. *Nursing Times*; 103(36):24–25.

Jevon P, Humphrey N (2007b) Respiratory procedures part 4: use of a spacer device. *Nursing Times*; 103(35):24–25.

McFerran T, Martin E (2003) *Mini-Dictionary for Nurses*, 5th edn. Oxford University Press, Oxford.

Müller M, Hänsel M, Stehr S *et al.* (2008) A state-wide survey of medical emergency management in dental practices: incidence of emergencies and training experience. *Emergency Medicine Journal*; 25:296–300.

Newell K, Hume S (2006) Choosing the right inhaler for patients with asthma. *Nursing Standard*; 21(5):46–48.

National Institute for Clinical Excellence (2004) *Chronic Obstructive Pulmonary Disease – Management of Chronic Obstructive Pulmonary Disease in Adults in Primary and Secondary Care*. NICE, London.

Pearce L (2000) Know How: Inhaler devices. *Nursing Times*; 96(37):16.

Rees J, Kanabar D (2007) *ABC of Asthma*, 5th edn. Blackwell Publishing, Oxford.

Resuscitation Council (UK) (2012) *Medical Emergencies and Resuscitation Standards for Clinical Practice and Training for Dental Practitioners and Dental Care Professionals in General Dental Practice*. Resuscitation Council (UK), London.

St John Ambulance, St Andrew's First Aid, British Red Cross (2011) *First Aid Manual*, Revised 9th edn. Dorling Kindersley, London.

Soanes C, Stevenson A (2006) *Oxford Dictionary of English*, 2nd edn. Oxford University Press, Oxford.

Sunderland R, Fleming M (2004) Continuing decline in acute asthma episodes in the community. *Archives of Disease in Childhood*; 89:282–285.

Ward J, Ward J, Leach R (2010) *The Respiratory System at a Glance*, 3rd edn. Wiley-Blackwell, Oxford.

Wyatt J, Illingworth R, Graham C et al (2012) *Oxford Handbook of Emergency Medicine* 4th edn. Oxford University Press, Oxford.

RESPIRATORY DISORDERS

Chapter 5
Cardiovascular disorders

INTRODUCTION

Cardiovascular disease (CVD) is the collective term for all diseases affecting the circulatory system (heart, arteries, blood vessels) (British Heart Foundation, 2012). In 2010, CVD were the United Kingdom's biggest killer: almost 180,000 people died from CVD, around 80,000 of these deaths being from coronary heart disease (CHD) and around 49,000 from strokes (British Heart Foundation, 2012). CVD causes around 46,000 premature deaths in the United Kingdom, 68% of which are in men (British Heart Foundation, 2012). Each year approximately 146,000 people suffer a myocardial infarction (MI; heart attack); one in three of these die before reaching hospital (British Heart Foundation, 2013). Chest pain, a characteristic symptom of CVD, is the commonest reason for alerting the emergency services; 10% of casualties taken to hospital with chest pain have had an acute MI (Laird *et al.*, 2004).

The aim of this chapter is to understand the management of cardiovascular disorders.

LEARNING OUTCOMES

At the end of the chapter the reader will be able to:

- Discuss the management of angina
- Discuss the management of a MI
- Discuss the management of palpitations
- Outlines the management of syncope

Basic Guide to Medical Emergencies in the Dental Practice, Second Edition. Phil Jevon.
© 2014 John Wiley & Sons, Ltd. Published 2014 by John Wiley & Sons, Ltd.
Companion website: www.wiley.com\go\jevon\medicalemergencies

MANAGEMENT OF ANGINA

Angina is a symptom of CHD. It is characterised by a heaviness or tightness in the centre of the chest that may spread to the arms, neck, jaw, face, back or stomach. Angina occurs when the arteries become so narrow that not enough oxygen-containing blood can reach the heart when its demands are high, such as during exercise (British Heart Foundation, 2012).

Angina is usually associated with risk factors including smoking, hypercholesterolaemia, hypertension, diabetes mellitus or a family history of ischaemic heart disease under the age of 60 years (Laird *et al.*, 2004).

In angina, the pain will ease with rest, though the administration of glyceryl trinitrate (GTN) spray or tablets may also be needed. Hospital admission is not necessary if the symptoms are mild and resolve with the patient's own medication (Resuscitation Council (UK), 2012; British Medical Association and Royal Pharmaceutical Society, 2012).

Patients diagnosed with angina, who are registered at the dental practice, should be asked to bring in their GTN with them when they attend for a check-up or treatment.

Precipitants

Precipitants of angina include:

- exercise, particularly climbing stairs or an incline;
- emotion, particularly anger or anxiety;
- a large meal – can increase cardiac output by 20%;
- cold, windy weather;
- exciting programmes on television – 'match of the day' angina;
- life-like, frightening dreams;
- sexual intercourse, particularly if extramarital or with a new partner.

Source: British Heart Foundation (2013)

In the dental practice, a patient with a history of angina could develop angina if he has to walk up some stairs to the surgery or if he is very stressed about having dental treatment.

Signs and symptoms

- A crushing pain, heaviness or tightness in the chest; or
- A pain in the arm, throat, neck, jaw, back or stomach;
- Sometimes the pain is associated with sweating, light-headedness, sickness or becoming short of breath.

Source: British Heart Foundation (2013)

CARDIOVASCULAR DISORDERS

Treatment

> If the patient has not been diagnosed with heart disease and has chest pain, it is recommended to call 999 immediately (British Heart Foundation, 2013 British Heart Foundation, 2009)

If a patient, who has already been diagnosed with CHD and has GTN spray or tablets, develops the above symptoms in the dental practice: often this will be angina that can be managed with rest and GTN, but it could be a MI (heart attack) (British Heart Foundation, 2013). The patient should be managed as follows (British Heart Foundation, 2013):

- Ask the patient to stop what he is doing or sit down and rest.
- Ask the patient to take his GTN spray or tablets (Figure 5.1) as prescribed by his general practitioner. It is recommended that the dental practice should stock GTN, in case the patient does not have his own GTN with him (Resuscitation Council (UK), 2012).
- If the pain has not eased within a few minutes, ask the patient to take a second dose.
- If, after the repeated dose, the pain does not ease within a few minutes, call 999 for an ambulance immediately. In addition, if the patient is not allergic to aspirin, administer 300 mg (ask him to chew it); this is administered for its anti-platelet effect (British Medical Association and Royal Pharmaceutical Society, 2012).

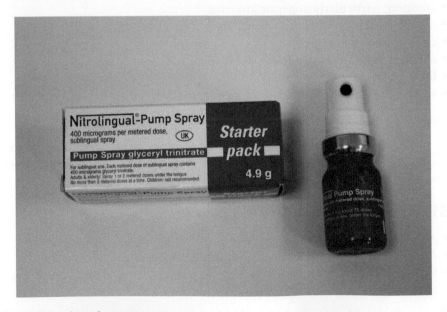

Figure 5.1 Glyceryl trinitrate spray.

- Even if the symptoms do not match the ones described above, but it is suspected that the patient is having a MI, call 999 for an ambulance immediately.

NB: Patients with known angina are usually asked to have their GTN spray easily accessible when attending for dental treatment.

MANAGEMENT OF MYOCARDIAL INFARCTION

Every 6 minutes someone dies from a heart attack
Every 11 minutes a man dies from a heart attack
Every 13 minutes a woman dies from a heart attack

Source: British Heart Foundation (2013).

In the United Kingdom alone, over 146,000 people each year have a MI (British Heart Foundation, 2013). MI is the leading cause of death in the United Kingdom (Wyatt *et al.*, 2012), accounting for 90,000 deaths each year (British Heart Foundation, 2013).

Of sudden cardiac deaths 50% occur within the first hour of onset, and 75% within three hours of onset, of an acute MI (Laird *et al.*, 2004). The most common cause of death is ventricular fibrillation (Jevon, 2009).

The risk of this, together with the life-saving benefits of coronary reperfusion therapy (usually percutaneous transluminal coronary angioplasty (PTCA)), reinforces the importance of ensuring that the dental practice dials 999 for an ambulance if a patient is suspected of having an MI (Jevon, 2006). Approximately 1.4 million people over the age of 35 years living in the United Kingdom have survived a heart attack (British Heart Foundation, 2013).

Aspirin 300 mg (Figure 5.2) is a key treatment therapy, particularly in the pre-hospital situation (NICE, 2010; St John Ambulance *et al.*, 2010; Resuscitation Council (UK), 2012; British Heart Foundation, 2013), as it reduces the incidence of coronary reocclusion following thrombolytic therapy, reducing the incidence of cardiac death. It should be administered as soon as possible as long as the patient is not allergic to it (NICE, 2010). If aspirin is chewed, it is absorbed more quickly than if it is swallowed, in the early stages of an acute MI (Resuscitation Council (UK), 2012).

Pathogenesis

An MI is usually caused by the rupture of an atheromatous plaque in a coronary artery (Chesebro *et al.*, 1997). Prior to rupture, the majority of these

CARDIOVASCULAR DISORDERS

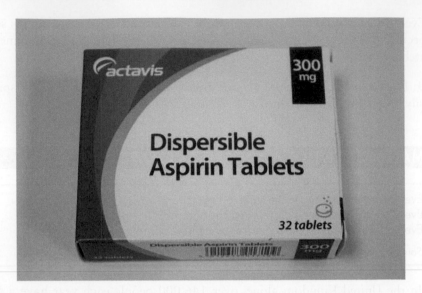

Figure 5.2 Aspirin 300 mg.

plaques are not haemodynamically significant (Ambrose and Fuster, 1997). However, once the plaque ruptures the following events are triggered:

- Haemorrhage into the plaque. This causes it to expand and restrict the lumen of the coronary artery;
- Contraction of the smooth muscle in the artery wall which will further restrict the lumen;
- Thrombus formation on the surface of the ruptured plaque (platelet adhesion) leading to total obstruction of the coronary lumen (Jevon, 2006).

Signs and symptoms
Common or typical symptoms include:

- Central chest pain;
- The pain can spread to the arms, neck or jaw;
- Feeling sick or sweaty as well as having central chest pain;
- Feeling short of breath as well as having central chest pain.

Symptoms vary and some people may feel any of the following:

- A dull pain, ache, or 'heavy' feeling in the chest;
- A mild discomfort in the chest making the patient feel generally unwell;
- The pain in the chest can spread to the back or stomach;
- A chest pain that feels like a bad episode of indigestion;
- Feeling a bit light-headed or dizzy as well as having chest pain.

Source: NICE (2010), British Heart Foundation (2013)

Sometimes the history can be unhelpful, e.g. a myocardial infarction may develop without any significant chest pain. Sometimes it is difficult to distinguish between cardiac and indigestion pains

Treatment

- If the patient displays the above symptoms and has not been diagnosed with heart disease, call 999 immediately (British Heart Foundation, 2013).
- Help the patient to adopt a relaxed position that reduces the myocardial workload: he will usually prefer to sit with his head and shoulders supported and his knees bent (Resuscitation Council (UK), 2012; British Heart Foundation, 2013) (Figure 5.3). Note: a supine position can sometimes provoke or worsen the pain. However, particularly if the patient is in shock, he may benefit from lying down (Resuscitation Council (UK), 2012).
- Reassure the patient and encourage him to rest.
- Offer the patient a single loading dose of 300 mg aspirin (crushed or chewed) as soon as possible unless there is clear evidence that they are allergic to it (if aspirin is given before arrival at hospital, send a written record with the person that it has been given) (NICE, 2010). The aspirin is administered for its anti-platelet effect (British Medical Association and Royal Pharmaceutical Society, 2012).

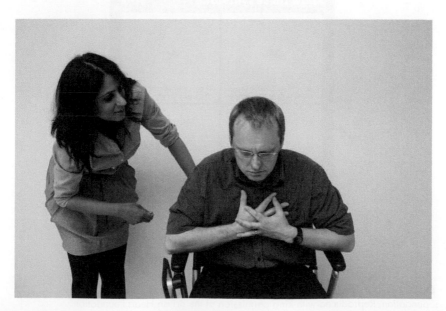

Figure 5.3 Sit the patient down (lay him flat if in shock).

CARDIOVASCULAR DISORDERS

- Offer the patient pain relief, e.g. GTN spray or tablets (NICE, 2010). Do warn the patient that side effects of GTN include a headache and light-headedness.
- Do not routinely administer oxygen (NICE, 2010). Administer high-flow oxygen (15 l/min) if the patient is cyanosed (blue lips) or conscious level deteriorates (Resuscitation Council (UK), 2012). If pulse oximetry is available (usually only in dental practices that use sedation), monitor oxygen saturation levels as soon as possible and only offer supplemental oxygen to patients with oxygen saturation (SpO_2) < 94% who are not at risk of hypercapnic respiratory failure, aiming for SpO_2 of 94–98% (in patients with chronic obstructive pulmonary disease (COPD) who are at risk of hypercapnic respiratory failure, administer oxygen to achieve a target SpO_2 of 88–92% (NICE, 2010).
- Closely monitor the patient; there is a risk of cardiopulmonary arrest.

There are many reasons why people delay calling 999 for an ambulance, e.g. uncertainty about the symptoms or not wishing to make a fuss (British Heart Foundation, 2013). The British Heart Foundation stress the importance of calling 999 (Figure 5.4)

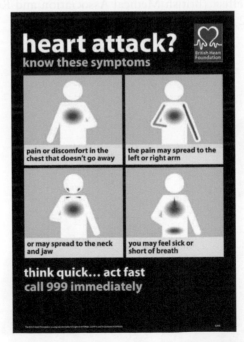

Figure 5.4 'Heart attack? Know these symptoms' poster. © 2014 British Heart Foundation. Reproduced with kind permission of the British Heart Foundation.

CARDIOVASCULAR DISORDERS

Once in hospital, patients may require percutaneous coronary intervention (PCI) – a minimally invasive approach to open narrowed coronary arteries (angioplasty) by accessing them through small needle-size punctures in the skin (British Heart Foundation, 2012). Angioplasty can be defined as a technique to widen a narrowed or obstructed blood vessel by inflating tightly folded balloons that have been passed into the narrowed location via a catheter. This technique squashes the fatty tissue that has caused the narrowing, hence widening the artery (British Heart Foundation, 2012).

MANAGEMENT OF PALPITATIONS

Palpitations are when the patient has a noticeable rapid, strong or irregular heartbeat (Soanes and Stevenson, 2006). Palpitations characteristically start and end abruptly.

Causes

Causes of palpitations include:

- ischaemic heart disease;
- drugs;
- tea or coffee;
- alcohol;
- stress.

Source: Jevon (2006)

Treatment

- Sit the patient down and ask him if he has had palpitations previously.
- Reassure the patient.
- Try vagal stimulation: the most effective way of doing this is a Valsalva manoeuvre (the action of attempting to exhale with the nostrils or mouth or glottis closed; Soanes and Stevenson, 2006) in the supine position (Wyatt *et al.*, 2012); ask the patient to cough or hold his nose and blow as if to pop his ears (Keech, 2004); another option is to ask the patient to attempt to blow the plunger out of a syringe (Figure 5.5) (impossible to do, but a safe effective vagal manoeuvre).
- If the patient is symptomatic, e.g. breathless, light-headed or has chest pain, call 999 for an ambulance; if the patient is not symptomatic, but the palpitations do not settle, seek medical advice (Keech, 2004).

Source: Jevon (2006)

CARDIOVASCULAR DISORDERS

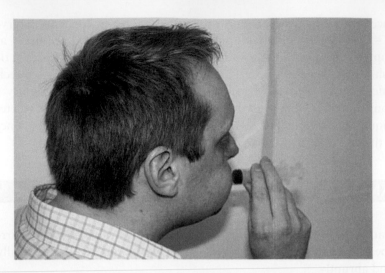

Figure 5.5 Example of a vagal manoeuvre: ask the patient to attempt to blow the plunger out of a syringe.

MANAGEMENT OF SYNCOPE

Syncope can be defined as a brief lapse in consciousness caused by transient reduction in blood flow to the brain (NICE, 2010). The term syncope derives from the Greek word meaning 'to cut short' (Soanes and Stevenson, 2006).

The commonest cause of syncope is a vasovagal attack or simple faint (British Medical Association and Royal Pharmaceutical Society, 2012). The term *vasovagal* relates to or denotes a temporary fall in blood pressure with pallor, fainting, sweating and nausea caused by overactivity of the vagus nerve, particularly as a result of stress (Soanes and Stevenson, 2006). Vasovagal syncope is the commonest medical emergency encountered in the dental practice, accounting for approximately two-thirds of all emergencies (Müller *et al.*, 2008).

It is estimated that 30% of the population have experienced a fainting episode and many more have observed friends or colleagues have one (Benditt and Goldstein, 2002).

Causes

Causes of syncope include:

• Emotional stress;
• Vagal stimulation;
• Vascular pooling in the legs (standing up for long periods);

- Diaphoresis (profuse sweating);
- Sudden change in environmental temperature;
- Sudden change in body position.

Source: NICE (2010)

Signs and symptoms

Signs and symptoms that may be evident include:

- sense of feeling unwell;
- light-headedness or dizziness;
- nausea and vomiting;
- sudden tiredness;
- yawning;
- blurred or tunnel vision;
- pallor;
- sudden collapse.

Source: Wyatt *et al.* (2012)

If the patient remains in an upright position, seizure-type twitching may occur (convulsive syncope) (Wyatt *et al.*, 2012).

Treatment

- If the patient feels faint, advise him to lie down; put the dental chair in a horizontal position. Raising the bottom end of the chair can be helpful.
- If the patient starts to collapse, if possible support him to the floor, taking care not to sustain an injury while doing so.
- Call out for help.
- Assess ABC to rule out cardiopulmonary arrest; as soon as the patient is horizontal he will usually start to regain consciousness.
- If the patient has collapsed on the floor, kneel down and raise his legs above the level of his heart (Figure 5.6).
- Ensure a supply of fresh air, e.g. loosen any light clothing around the neck and chest, open a nearby window or door and ask colleagues not to crowd around the patient.
- Reassure the patient.
- Check for any injuries; if the patient collapses during a faint, injuries, e.g. bone fractures or a head injury could be sustained, particularly in the elderly (Benditt and Goldstein, 2002).
- Note the duration of the syncope episode; if a simple faint, the patient will quickly recover, usually within 60 seconds (Benditt and Goldstein, 2002).

CARDIOVASCULAR DISORDERS

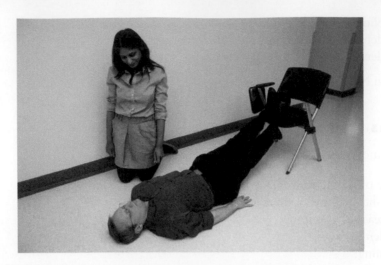

Figure 5.6 Dealing with a faint: lay the patient flat and raise the legs.

- Once the patient regains consciousness, offer a drink, e.g. sugar in water or a cup of sweet tea (British Medical Association and Royal Pharmaceutical Society, 2012).
- If the patient takes time to recover, place him in the recovery position. Assess the patient following the ABCDE approach. It may be necessary to call 999 for an ambulance.

Other considerations

- Always distinguish between an innocent 'simple faint' and a collapse due to a more sinister reason, e.g. a seizure or a cardiac event (Wyatt *et al.*, 2012). Cyanosis, tongue biting, saliva frothing at the mouth or incontinence suggest a generalised seizure (Wyatt *et al.*, 2012).
- Note any neurological signs during the episode (Wyatt *et al.*, 2012).
- Advise the patient to recognise and avoid situations that could cause him to faint (Benditt and Goldstein, 2002).

CONCLUSION

CVD are a leading cause of death in the United Kingdom. Chest pain, a characteristic symptom of cardiovascular disease, is the commonest reason for alerting the emergency services. In this chapter, the management of angina and MI have been discussed in detail. The management of palpitations and syncope have also been outlined.

REFERENCES

Ambrose J, Fuster V (1997) Can we predict future acute coronary events in patients with stable coronary artery disease?. *Journal of the American Medical Association*; 277:343–344.

Benditt D, Goldstein M (2002) Fainting. *Circulation*; 106:1048–1050.

British Heart Foundation (2013) www.bhf.org.uk (accessed 13 March 2013).

British Heart Foundation (2012) *Coronary Heart Disease Statistics 2012*, British Heart Foundation, London.

British Medical Association and Royal Pharmaceutical Society of Great Britain (2012) *British National Formulary 64*. BMJ Publishing, London.

Chesebro J, Rauch U, Fuster V, Badimon J (1997) Pathogenesis of thrombosis in coronary artery disease. *Haemostasis*; 27(suppl 1):12–18.

Jevon P (2006) *Emergency Care and First Aid for Nurses*. Elsevier, Oxford.

Jevon P (2009) *Advanced Cardiac Life Support*, 2nd edn. Wiley-Blackwell, Oxford.

Keech P (2004) *Practical Guide to First Aid*. Lorenz Books, London.

Laird C, Driscoll P, Wardrope J (2004) The ABC of community emergency care. 3 Chest pain. *Emergency Medicine Journal*; 21: 226–232.

Müller M, Hänsel M, Stehr S *et al.* (2008) A state-wide survey of medical emergency management in dental practices: incidence of emergencies and training experience. *Emergency Medicine Journal*; 25: 296–300.

NICE (2010) http://guidance.nice.org.uk/CG95 (accessed 02 October 2013).

Resuscitation Council (UK) (2012) *Medical Emergencies and Resuscitation Standards for Clinical Practice and Training for Dental Practitioners and Dental Care Professionals in General Dental Practice*. Resuscitation Council (UK), London.

Soanes C, Stevenson A (2006) *Oxford Dictionary of English*, 2nd edn. Oxford University Press, Oxford.

St John Ambulance, St Andrews Ambulance Association & British Red Cross (2010) *First Aid Manual* Dorling Kindersley, London.

Wyatt J, Illingworth R, Graham C *et al.* (2012) *Oxford Handbook of Emergency Medicine*, 4th edn. Oxford University Press, Oxford.

CARDIOVASCULAR DISORDERS

Chapter 6

Endocrine disorders

INTRODUCTION

Endocrine disorders account for approximately 1.5% of all hospital emergency admissions in England; the majority are related to diabetes (Kearney and Dang, 2007). In the dental practice, hypoglycaemia is by far the most likely endocrine disorder to be encountered. Adrenal insufficiency may also occur.

The aim of this chapter is to understand the management of endocrine disorders.

LEARNING OUTCOMES

At the end of this chapter the reader will be able to:

- Discuss the management of hypoglycaemia
- Describe the procedure for blood glucose measurement using a glucometer
- Discuss the management of adrenal insufficiency

MANAGEMENT OF HYPOGLYCAEMIA

Hypoglycaemia is normally defined as a blood glucose level < 3 mmol/L (Resuscitation Council (UK), 2012) and is usually associated with diabetes (particularly patients taking insulin). When attending for dental treatment, diabetic patients should eat as normal and should take their medication, e.g. insulin or oral hypoglycaemic agent, as prescribed (Resuscitation Council (UK), 2012; British Medical Association and Royal Pharmaceutical Society, 2012). If a meal is missed, then hypoglycaemia can occur (British Medical Association and Royal Pharmaceutical Society, 2012).

Basic Guide to Medical Emergencies in the Dental Practice, Second Edition. Phil Jevon.
© 2014 John Wiley & Sons, Ltd. Published 2014 by John Wiley & Sons, Ltd.
Companion website: www.wiley.com\go\jevon\medicalemergencies

Incidence

The exact incidence of hypoglycaemic episodes in the general population is unknown, as most are treated successfully at home and some, particularly those occurring at night, may not even be recognised. On average there are over 90,000 calls to the emergency services each year for hypoglycaemia (Sampson *et al.*, 2006). In 2004/5 there were 8000 admissions to hospital in England due to hypoglycaemia (Kearney and Dang, 2007).

Hypoglycaemia accounts for approximately 22% of medical emergencies encountered in the dental surgery (Müller *et al.*, 2008). Diabetic patients treated with insulin are most likely to become hypoglycaemic while attending for dental treatment (Resuscitation Council (UK), 2012).

Risks

The risks associated with hypoglycaemia are small, though altered level of consciousness can always lead to airway compromise. However, hypoglycaemia can cause an acute cerebral injury, leading to hemiplegia (Shirayama *et al.*, 2004); a prolonged severe hypoglycaemic episode can even cause moderate to severe neuropsychological impairments (Kubiak *et al.*, 2004).

Causes of hypoglycaemia

Common causes of hypoglycaemia include:

- too much insulin;
- delayed or missed meal or snack;
- insufficient food, especially carbohydrate;
- unplanned or strenuous exercise;
- alcohol consumption without food;
- idiopathic.

Source: Diabetes UK (2013)

Medical causes of hypoglycaemia include:

- liver failure;
- Addison's disease;
- pituitary insufficiency.

Source: Wyatt *et al.* (2012)

Nearly all hypoglycaemic episodes occur in patients who are prescribed insulin treatment, though episodes may rarely occur in patients prescribed sulphonylurea drugs (Shorr *et al.*, 1997); these drugs, e.g. glibenclamide, augment insulin production (British Medical Association and Royal Pharmaceutical Society, 2012).

ENDOCRINE DISORDERS

Consumption of alcohol can lead to hypoglycaemia several hours later; in addition, the effects of alcohol can mask the symptoms of hypoglycaemia.

Clinical features

The clinical features of hypoglycaemia vary from person to person, though they are often constant for an individual (Diabetes UK, 2013). Individuals may recognise different symptoms and these may change as the duration of diabetes increases (McLaren and Somerville, 1988).

Clinical features of hypoglycaemia can be classified as either autonomic (usually present first when the blood glucose is 3.3–3.6 mmol/L) or related to neuroglycopenia (usually present when the blood glucose is less than 2.6 mmol/L):

- *Autonomic:* sweating, hunger, hot sensation, anxiety, nausea and vomiting;
- *Neuroglycopenia:* fatigue, visual disturbance, uncoordinated and altered behaviour, drowsiness, confusion and if untreated convulsions and coma. (Turner and Wass, 2009; British Medical Association and Royal Pharmaceutical Society, 2012; Diabetes UK, 2013).

NB: in patients with chronic hyperglycaemia, the autonomic clinical features may be triggered at higher blood glucose levels.

Hypoglycaemia is a recognized complication of insulin therapy; at the onset most patients recognize the symptoms and are able to take remedial action but this hypoglycaemia awareness decreases over time so much so that after 20 years of insulin treatment 50% of these patients are unaware of their symptoms (Greenstein and Wood, 2011). The dental practitioner should therefore always be alert to the clinical features of hypoglycaemia.

Diagnosis

Ideally blood glucose measurement should be undertaken in the dental practice. It is recommended that each dental practice has an automated blood glucose measurement device (Resuscitation Council (UK), 2012). The biomedical diagnosis of hypoglycaemia is a blood sugar less than 3.0 mmol/L (Resuscitation Council (UK), 2012). A suggested procedure for blood glucose measurement is described in Chapter 3.

Treatment

- Assess the patient following the ABCDE approach described in Chapter 3. Treatment will depend upon the patient's level of consciousness and degree of co-operation (Wyatt *et al.*, 2012; Resuscitation Council (UK), 2012).

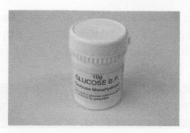

Figure 6.1 Glucose 10 mg.

- If the patient's consciousness level allows him to safely eat and drink, offer him the simplest available and quickly absorbed food or drink that contains carbohydrate, e.g. a glass of Lucozade or cola (not diet drinks), a glass of fruit juice, or 3–4 glucose tablets (Diabetes UK, 2013). Repeat this after 10–15 minutes if necessary (British Medical Association and Royal Pharmaceutical Society, 2012).
- Following initial treatment, offer the patient a snack providing sustained availability of carbohydrate, e.g. sandwich, fruit, milk or biscuits, or the next meal if it is due, to help prevent the blood-glucose concentration from falling again (British Medical Association and Royal Pharmaceutical Society, 2012).
- GlucoGel (Figure 6.1; formerly known as Hypostop), a dextrose gel stocked in most dental surgeries, is rapidly absorbed via the buccal mucosa. GlucoGel or similar may be administered (British Medical Association and Royal Pharmaceutical Society, 2012; Kearney and Dang, 2007).

In more severe cases, where the patient's level of consciousness deteriorates:

- Ensure his airway is clear and maintained; place him in the lateral position. If he is unconscious consider inserting a basic airway device, e.g. oropharyngeal airway (see Chapter 10).
- Administer high flow oxygen using a non-rebreathe mask (see Chapter 10). If available, attach pulse oximetry to monitor oxygen saturation.
- Administer glucagon 1 mg (Figure 6.2) IM/SC (hormone produced by the A-cells of the islets in the pancreas); it increases the blood glucose level by mobilising glycogen stores in the liver. The majority of people with type 1 diabetes lose their glucagon response to hypoglycaemia within 5 years of diagnosis

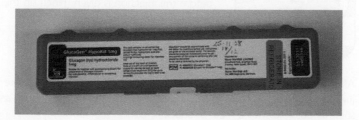

Figure 6.2 Glucagon.

ENDOCRINE DISORDERS

(Bolli *et al.*, 1983). The recommended dose for glucagon is 1 mg subcutaneously or intramuscularly (British Medical Association & Royal Pharmaceutical Society, 2012). The procedure for administering glucagon is described in Box 6.1.

Box 6.1 Procedure for administering glucagon. With kind permission from Novo Nordisk Ltd.

Using GlucaGen®HypoKit Step by Step Guide

Instructions for use

1. Remove the orange plastic cap of the GlucaGen bottle. Insert the needle through the rubber seal disk on the bottle. Inject all the liquid in the syringe into the bottle. The rubber seal can be stiff, but the needle is strong enough to puncture it.

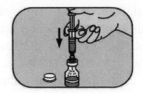

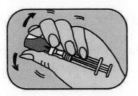

2. Leave the syringe in place and gently shake the bottle until the powder is completely dissolved, and the solution is clear.

3. Make sure the plunger is totally down, then gently pull it out until all the solution is drawn up into the syringe.

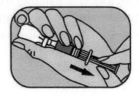

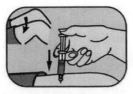

4. Ensure that there is no air in the syringe, before the injection is given. Pinch up the skin and inject the needle into it, for example in the outer thigh. You cannot harm the person by giving this injection.

5. After the injection, when the person responds, give a sweet drink like juice or a soft drink, to keep blood glucose levels up. Follow this up as soon as possible with a meal or snack.

- Monitor the patient's response and level of consciousness; 90% of patients will fully recover in 20 minutes (Wyatt *et al.*, 2012).
- If able, recheck the blood glucose after 10 minutes to ensure that it has improved (5 mmol/L or more), in conjunction with an improvement in the patient's level of consciousness and AVPU scale (Resuscitation Council (UK), 2012).
- Try to establish the possible cause of the hypoglycaemia. To prevent a repeat hypoglycaemic episode, offer the patient food that contains starchy carbohydrates (absorbed more slowly), e.g. a sandwich, fruit or biscuits and milk (Diabetes (UK), 2013).
- Educate the patient. Education is the key to preventing recurrent or severe hypoglycaemia. It may be necessary to advise the patient to make an appointment to go to see his GP or practice nurse for assessment and advice.
- Reassure the patient. Repeated episodes of hypoglycaemia may cause extreme emotional distress, even when the episodes are relatively mild.
- If it was necessary to administer glucagon to the patient, he may go home once fully recovered, but should be accompanied; he should not drive and his GP should be informed (Resuscitation Council (UK), 2012).

When to call 999 for an ambulance

For some patients with hypoglycaemia, it will definitely be necessary to call 999 for an ambulance, particularly if the cause is an oral anti-diabetic drug because the hypoglycaemic effects of the drug may last for several hours (British Medical Association and Royal Pharmaceutical Society, 2012).

PROCEDURE FOR BLOOD GLUCOSE MEASUREMENT USING A GLUCOMETER

The procedure for blood glucose measurement involves obtaining a small sample of the patient's blood, usually from his fingertip, and applying it to a test strip inserted into an electronic meter (glucometer) (Figure 6.3). The result

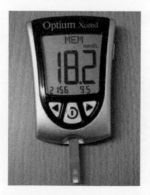

Figure 6.3 Blood glucose measurement device or glucometer.

is expressed in millimoles per litre (mmol/L), i.e. it is a measurement of millimoles of glucose per litre of blood. It is recommended that a glucometer should be available in the dental practice (Resuscitation Council (UK), 2012).

Indications

In the dental practice, it would be helpful to undertake blood glucose measurement if hypoglycaemia (see Chapter 3) is suspected, or after a seizure (Resuscitation Council (UK), 2012).

Procedure

Described below is a typical procedure for blood glucose measurement using a glucometer device. It is important to follow the manufacturer's recommendations for the specific device being used in the dental practice.

- Explain the procedure to the patient.
- Assemble equipment: glucometer (ensure that a high/low test has been done as recommended by the manufacturer), finger-prick device, sharps box, test strip (ensure it is in date and matches the calibration code for the glucometer), gauze swab or similar.
- Wash and dry your hands and don gloves.
- Discuss the procedure with the patient – he may be able to advise on his normal blood glucose measurement and also on the best site to obtain the blood sample from. It would be helpful to choose an alternative site to one which was last used (the skin can become sore).
- Ensure that the finger being used is clean and dry (dirt contamination could affect the result).
- Using the finger-prick device, stab the side of the finger (less painful than the centre) to draw blood (Figure 6.4) and dispose of the sharp safely in the sharps box.

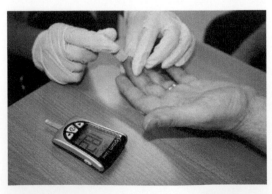

Figure 6.4 Blood glucose measurement: using the finger-prick device, stab the side of the finger.

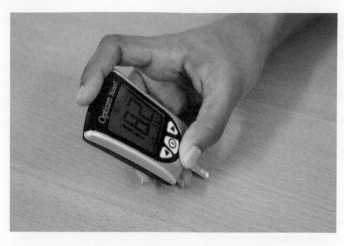

Figure 6.5 Blood glucose measurement: wait for the reading to be displayed on the glucometer.

- Allow a droplet of blood to form (gentle squeezing may be necessary) onto the test strip following the manufacturer's recommendations.
- Apply gauze to puncture site and press to stop the bleeding; some patients will like a plaster, some will not.
- Wait for the reading to be displayed on the glucometer (Figure 6.5), documenting the result.

MANAGEMENT OF ADRENAL INSUFFICIENCY

Adrenal insufficiency is a potentially fatal condition resulting from inadequate secretion of cortisol and/or aldosterone (Boon *et al.*, 2006). It can be associated with prolonged corticosteroid therapy and can persist for years after stopping. A patient with adrenal insufficiency, when attending for dental treatment, may become very stressed, which could lead to hypotension and shock (British Medical Association and Royal Pharmaceutical Society, 2012).

Causes

Adrenal insufficiency can result from:

- *Primary adrenal insufficiency:* results from adrenal damage, e.g. Addison's disease;
- *Secondary adrenal insufficiency:* results from adrenocorticotrophic hormone (ACTH) deficiency due to pituitary or hypothalamic damage;

ENDOCRINE DISORDERS

- Abrupt withdrawal of therapeutic steroid therapy can also cause ACTH deficiency;
- Stress, e.g. attending for dental treatment.

Clinical features

Clinical features include:

- shock, e.g. hypotension, tachycardia and pallor;
- anorexia;
- nausea and vomiting;
- abdominal pain;
- pyrexia;
- fatigue and lethargy.

Source: Kearney and Dang (2007)

Treatment

- Assess the patient following the ABCDE approach described in Chapter 3.
- Call 999 for an ambulance.
- Lie the patient flat in the dental chair.
- Administer high flow oxygen using a non-rebreathe mask (see Chapter 3). If available, establish oxygen saturation monitoring using a pulse oximeter.

CONCLUSION

Endocrine disorders can be encountered in the dental practice. The management of hypoglycaemia in the dental practice has been discussed including blood glucose measurement. The management of the adrenal insufficiency has also been outlined.

REFERENCES

Bolli G, De Feo P, Compagnucci P *et al.* (1983) Abnormal glucose counter-regulation in insulin-dependent diabetes mellitus: interaction of anti-insulin antibodies and impaired glucagon and epinephrine secretion. *Diabetes*; 32:134–141.

Boon N, Colledge N, Walker B, Hunter J (2006) *Davidson's Principles & Practice of Medicine*, 20th edn. Churchill Livingstone, Edinburgh.

British Medical Association & Royal Pharmaceutical Society of Great Britain (2012) *BNF 64*. BMJ Publishing, London.

Diabetes UK (2013) www.diabetes.org.uk (accessed 4 April 2013).

Greenstein B, Wood D (2011) *The Endocrine System at a Glance,* 3rd edn. Wiley, London.

Kearney T, Dang C (2007) Diabetic and endocrine emergencies. *Postgraduate Medical Journal;* 83(976):79–86.

Kubiak T, Kuhr B, Inselmann D, *et al.* (2004) Reversible cognitive deterioration after a single episode of severe hypoglycaemia. *Diabetic Medicine;* 21:1366–1367.

McLaren E, Somerville J (1988) Early warning symptoms of hypoglycaemia in ambulant diabetics. *Practical Diabetes;* 5:207–208.

Müller M, Hänsel M, Stehr S *et al.* (2008) A state-wide survey of medical emergency management in dental practices: incidence of emergencies and training experience. *Emergency Medicine Journal;* 25:296–300.

Resuscitation Council (UK) (2012) *Medical emergencies and resuscitation – standards for clinical practice and training for dental practitioners and dental care professionals in general dental practice.* Resuscitation Council (UK), London.

Sampson M, Mortley S, Aldridge V (2006) The East Anglian Ambulance Trust diabetes emergencies audit: numbers and demographics. *Diabetes Medicine;* 23:101.

Shirayama H, Ohshiro Y, Kinjo Y *et al.* (2004) Acute brain injury in hypoglycaemia-induced hemiplegia. *Diabetic Medicine;* 21:623–624.

Shorr R, Ray W, Daugherty J *et al.* (1997) Incidence and risk factors for serious hypoglycaemia in older persons using insulin or sulfonylureas. *Archives of Internal Medicine;* 157;1681–1686.

Turner H, Wass J (2009) *Oxford Handbook of Endocrinology and Diabetes,* 2nd edn. Oxford University Press, Oxford.

Wyatt J, Illingworth R, Graham C *et al.* (2012) *Oxford Handbook of Emergency Medicine,* 4th edn. Oxford University Press, Oxford.

ENDOCRINE DISORDERS

Chapter 7

Neurological disorders

INTRODUCTION

Neurological disorders account for approximately 20% of admissions to general hospitals in the United Kingdom, an increasing proportion of which are emergencies (Sharief and Anand, 1997). Neurological disorders can be life threatening; altered consciousness level can lead to a compromised airway and compromised breathing. Neurological disorders in the dental practice require prompt effective treatment, together with close monitoring of ABCDE to detect deterioration.

The aim of this chapter is to understand the management of neurological disorders.

LEARNING OUTCOMES

At the end of this chapter the reader will be able to:

- Discuss the management of a generalised tonic–clonic seizure
- Discuss the management of a stroke
- Discuss the management of altered level of consciousness
- Describe the procedure for placing a patient in the recovery position

MANAGEMENT OF A GENERALISED TONIC–CLONIC SEIZURE

A seizure happens when there is a sudden burst of intense electrical activity in the brain (often referred to as epileptic activity), causing a temporary disruption to the way the brain normally works, resulting in an epileptic seizure

Basic Guide to Medical Emergencies in the Dental Practice, Second Edition. Phil Jevon.
© 2014 John Wiley & Sons, Ltd. Published 2014 by John Wiley & Sons, Ltd.
Companion website: www.wiley.com\go\jevon\medicalemergencies

(Epilepsy Action, 2013). In the United Kingdom, 600,000 people have epilepsy (Epilepsy Action, 2013). The incidence of epilepsy is estimated to be 50 per 100,000 per year and the prevalence of active epilepsy in the United Kingdom is estimated to be 5–10 cases per 1000 (NICE, 2012). Two-thirds of people with active epilepsy have their epilepsy controlled satisfactorily with anti-epileptic drugs (NICE, 2012).

There are over 40 different types of seizures; a person may have more than one type and recurrent seizures are defined as epilepsy (Epilepsy Action, 2013). In this section, the management of a patient having a generalised tonic–clonic seizure, sometimes called a grand mal fit, will be discussed. In the dental practice, these seizures account for approximately 7% of all medical emergencies encountered in the dental surgery (Müller *et al.*, 2008).

Sudden unexpected death in epilepsy accounts for approximately 500 deaths each year (National Institute for Clinical Excellence (NICE), 2002). Status epilepticus, a potentially life-threatening medical emergency, is associated with significant morbidity and mortality if not treated promptly (NICE, 2002). Injuries that can be sustained include fractures, burns, dislocations, concussion and intracerebral haemorrhage (American Heart Association, 2005). Dental injuries are quite common (Buck *et al.*, 1997). Maintaining the patient's safety during a seizure is a priority.

Signs and symptoms

Typical characteristics of a generalised tonic–clonic seizure (Jevon, 2006; Turner, 2007; Epilepsy Action, 2013; St John Ambulance *et al.*, 2011) include:

- Sudden loss of consciousness (can be preceded by crying out) and collapse to the ground;
- Rigidity (tonic phase) – lasting for approximately 10 seconds, the body is stiff, the elbows are flexed and the legs are extended;
- Breathing stops; central cyanosis particularly noticeable around the mouth;
- Clenching of the jaw – saliva may accumulate at the mouth, which could be blood-stained if the casualty has bitten his tongue or lip;
- Convulsive movements (clonic phase) – lasting for 1–2 minutes, there is violent generalised rhythmical shaking;
- Incontinence;
- Variable period of unconsciousness following the event. The casualty may feel very tired and may fall into a deep sleep; he could be dazed, confused, disorientated, frightened and may have slurred, incomprehensible speech.

Causes

Causes of a generalised tonic–clonic seizure include:

- epilepsy (most common cause);
- head injury;
- certain poisons, e.g. alcohol, ecstasy;
- alcohol withdrawal;
- cerebral hypoxia;
- cerebral hypoglycaemia (Jevon, 2006).

Treatment

- If necessary, call 999 for an ambulance (see later in When to call 999 for an ambulance).
- Ensure that it is safe to approach the patient.
  - Ask other patients to leave the room.
- Protect the patient from injury. Ensure the space around him is clear and remove any objects that are potentially dangerous objects.
- Loosen any clothing around the patient's neck.
- Cushion the patient's head, e.g. place something soft such as a pillow, jumper or jacket under his head. Alternatively, place the palms of your hands behind his head and support it to prevent injury.
- Administer oxygen 15 l/min.
  - Note the time in order to check how long the seizure lasts.
  - Consider measuring the patient's blood glucose (fitting can be a presenting sign of hypoglycaemia), particularly if the patient is a child or a known diabetic (Resuscitation Council (UK), 2012). Treat hypoglycaemia if present (see pages).
- Check to see if the patient has a very slow pulse (<40 per minute) because this can lead to hypotension (low blood pressure) which can cause transient cerebral hypoxia leading to a brief seizure (Resuscitation Council (UK), 2012).
- Administer midazolam 10 mg via the buccal route (Figure 7.1) if seizures are prolonged (5 minutes or longer) or if the seizures are repeated rapidly (Resuscitation Council (UK), 2012; NICE, 2012) (British Medical Association and Royal Pharmaceutical Society, 2013) (the doses of buccal midazolam in children are <5 years – 5 mg; 5–10 years – 7.5 mg; >10 years – 10 mg). There are currently three midazolam presentations listed in the latest BNF for buccal use (British Medical Association and Royal Pharmaceutical Society of Great Britain, 2013): midazolam injection (unlicensed), epistatus (unlicensed) and buccolam (paediatric licence; unlicensed in adults). In the dental practice, midazolam should be administered by (or under the supervision of) a dental practitioner (Resuscitation Council (UK), 2012).

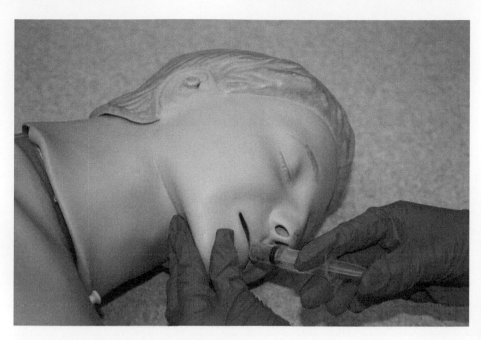

Figure 7.1 Buccal administration of midazolam.

NEUROLOGICAL DISORDERS

- Once the seizure has stopped continue to monitor airway, breathing and circulation; if the patient is breathing normally, place him in the recovery position (if the patient is not breathing normally, start resuscitation – see Chapter 9).
- Wipe away any saliva; suction may be necessary.
- Check to see whether the patient has sustained any injuries.
- Calmly reassure the patient.
- Stay with the patient until he has made a complete recovery.
- Continue to administer oxygen to support breathing if necessary.

Source: St John Ambulance *et al.* (2011), Jevon and Morgan (2007), Epilepsy Action (2013), National Society for Epilepsy (2013)

> Buccal midazolam is the first-line treatment in children, young people and adults with prolonged (lasting 5 minutes or more) or repeated (three or more in an hour) seizures in the community (NICE, 2012)

When to call 999 for an ambulance

Call 999 for an ambulance if:

- it is the patient's first seizure; or
- the seizure continues for longer than 5 minutes; or
- one tonic–clonic seizure follows another without the casualty regaining consciousness between seizures (status epilepticus); or
- the patient incurs an injury during the seizure; or
- the patient requires urgent medical attention; or
- there is difficulty monitoring the patient; or
- there is a high risk of recurrence.

Source: NICE (2012), Resuscitation Council (UK) (2012)

Action not recommended during a seizure

During a seizure it is recommended not to:

- Restrain the patient;
- Insert anything in the patient's mouth;
- Move the patient unless he is in danger;
- Give the patient anything to eat or drink until he has fully recovered;
- Attempt to arouse the patient.

Source: Epilepsy Action (2013)

Observations during a seizure

'A clear history from the casualty and an eyewitness to the attack give the most important diagnostic information, and should be the mainstay of diagnosis' (Scottish Intercollegiate Guidelines Network, 2003). The following observations during a seizure will assist in its diagnosis and classification:

- Where was the patient and what was he doing prior to the seizure?
- Any mood change, e.g. excitement, anger or anxiety?
- Unusual sensations, e.g. odd smell or taste?
- Any prior warning?

- Loss of consciousness or confusion?
- Any colour change, e.g. pallor, cyanosis? If so where, e.g. face, lips, hand?
- Altered respiratory pattern, e.g. dyspnoea, noising respirations?
- Which part of the body affected by seizure?
- Incontinence?
- Tongue biting?
- Did the patient do anything unusual, e.g. mumble, wander about or fumble with his clothing?
- How long did the seizure last?
- How was the patient following the seizure? Did the patient need to sleep and, if so, for how long?
- How long before the patient can perform normal activities again?

Source: National Society for Epilepsy (2013)

Personalized care plane

A patient with epilepsy may have a personalised care plan drawn up by the local hospital which will probably include action in the event of a seizure. Although it would be prudent to follow this care plan should the patient have a seizure in the dental practice. However, it is still important to call 999 for an ambulance if it is indicated (see When to call 999 for an ambulance section in this chapter).

MANAGEMENT OF STROKE

A stroke can be defined as a sudden onset of neurological impairment that is caused by a disruption of the blood supply to the brain with symptoms lasting > 24 hours (Mant and Walker, 2011). A stroke is a medical emergency; each year 150,000 people in the UK have a stroke, most of whom are over 65 years of age (Stroke Association, 2013). Stroke is the third biggest cause of death and the single most common cause of disability in the UK (Stroke Association, 2013). A patient suffering a stroke requires immediate treatment, which is directed towards sustaining life and preventing further brain damage (Mant and Walker, 2011).

A transient ischaemic attack (TIA), sometimes called a mini-stroke, is when the brain's blood supply is interrupted for a brief time; although the symptoms are similar to a stroke they are only temporary, lasting minutes or hours but disappearing completely within 24 hours (Stroke Association, 2013). A transient ischaemic attack could lead to a major stroke: the patient should be reviewed by his GP as soon as possible and referred to a specialist stroke service within 7 days (Stroke Association, 2013).

NEUROLOGICAL DISORDERS

Pathogenesis

A stroke is caused by either cerebral infarction or cerebral haemorrhage:

- *Cerebral infarction (80%):* due to thrombosis, cerebral embolism (e.g. from atrial fibrillation or valve disease/replacement) or very occasionally an episode of hypoperfusion;
- *Cererbral haemorrhage (20%):* associated with hypertension, subarachnoid haemorrhage and bleeding disorders.

Source: Wyatt *et al.* (2012)

Symptoms

The symptoms will depend on the type of stroke, the area affected and the extent of the stroke. Symptoms may include:

- sudden weakness or numbness of the face, arm or leg on one side of the body;
- sudden severe unexplained headache;
- sudden loss or blurring of vision, in one or both eyes;
- sudden difficulty in speaking or understanding spoken language;
- sudden confusion;
- loss of balance – dizziness, unsteadiness or a sudden fall, particularly with any of the above signs.

Source: Stroke Association (2013)

Recognition of a stroke: FAST

The Stroke Association (2013) recommends following the FAST (Figure 7.2) approach when assessing whether a patient has had a stroke:

- *Facial weakness:* can the patient smile? Has her mouth or an eye drooped?
- *Arm weakness:* can the patient raise both arms?
- *Speech problems:* can the patient speak clearly and understand what is being said to him?
- *Test all three symptoms.*

These simple checks can help to ascertain whether the patient has had a stroke or not.

Treatment

- Assess the patient following the ABCDE approach described in chapter 3. Also assess the patient following the FAST approach (see above); if a stroke is suspected call 999 for an ambulance (Stroke Association, 2013).

NEUROLOGICAL DISORDERS

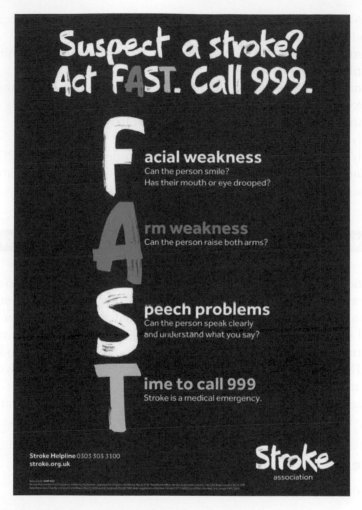

Figure 7.2 The Stroke Association's FAST guidelines for assessing a patient with a suspected stroke. *Source:* The Stroke Association. Reproduced with permission.

- Ensure the patient has a clear airway. Following a stroke the airway can become compromised by the tongue and/or secretions in the mouth. Ensure the patient's airway remains patent: aspiration of gastric contents or secretions is a serious complication of a stroke, which is associated with considerable morbidity and mortality (American Heart Association, 2005).
- If the patient is unconscious (but breathing normally), place him in the recovery position; inserting an oropharyngeal airway may be helpful.
- If the patient is conscious, ensure his head and shoulders are supported in a slightly raised position, thus helping to protect the airway; tilting the head towards the affected side allows secretions to drain out; wipe the mouth with

a flannel or similar (St John Ambulance *et al.*, 2011). It may be necessary to suction the mouth.

- Regularly monitor the patient's airway and do not give him anything to eat or drink (Wyatt *et al.*, 2012).
- Administer high flow oxygen using a non-rebreathe mask. If available, establish oxygen saturation monitoring using a pulse oximeter. Closely monitor the patient's breathing as ventilatory support may be required.
- Closely monitor the patient's vital signs.
- Closely monitor the patient's level of consciousness, using the AVPU scale.
- Reassure the patient. Once the patient regains consciousness the patient may be disorientated and may have a headache requiring analgesia.

MANAGEMENT OF ALTERED LEVEL OF CONSCIOUSNESS

The patient's level of consciousness has been described as the degree of his arousal and awareness (Geraghty, 2005). It is dependent upon the interaction of the ascending reticular activating system situated in the brainstem and the cerebral hemispheres (Jevon and Morgan, 2007). Any disruption in this communication process will result in altered consciousness (Bassett and Makin, 2000). The manifestation of altered consciousness implies an underlying brain dysfunction (Geraghty, 2005).

The term 'unconsciousness' can be defined as not awake, not aware of and not responding to one's environment (Soanes and Stevenson, 2006).

Causes

Causes of altered level of consciousness include:

- metabolic disturbances, e.g. hypoglycaemia, hypothyroidism;
- trauma, e.g. head injury;
- stroke;
- infection, e.g. meningitis;
- drugs, e.g. opiates, midazolam;
- alcohol.

Source: Jevon (2006)

Investigations

While awaiting the arrival of an ambulance, it would help to try to establish the possible cause of the unconsciousness, e.g. if able, check the patient's blood sugar for the presence of hypoglycaemia.

Treatment

> If the patient appears to be unconscious and lifeless, follow the resuscitation protocols described in chapter 9 and start cardiopulmonary resuscitation immediately if required

Review ABCDE

- Assess the patient following the ABCDE approach described in chapter 3. As a compromised airway, inadequate breathing or inadequate circulation can lead to altered conscious level, attention to these is a priority (Wyatt *et al.*, 2012).
- If necessary, call 999 for an ambulance.
- Ensure the patient has a clear airway. The airway can become compromised by the tongue and/or secretions, vomit, etc. in the mouth. If the patient is unconscious (but breathing), place in the recovery position (see below) and consider inserting an oropharyngeal airway (see pages). Regular oral suction may be required. If the patient has dentures, these are usually only removed if they are loose or ill-fitting.
- Regularly monitor the patient's airway (Wyatt *et al.*, 2012).
- If necessary administer oxygen. If available, establish oxygen saturation monitoring using a pulse oximeter. Closely monitor the patient's respiratory rate as ventilatory support may be required.
- Closely monitor the patient's level of consciousness, using the AVPU scale, and undertake regular assessment of the pupils.
- If able, perform blood glucose measurement. Treat confirmed or suspected hypoglycaemia.
- Check the patient's medication history for recent administration of a mediation that may cause unconsciousness, e.g. an opiate.

PROCEDURE FOR PLACING A PATIENT IN THE RECOVERY POSITION

In an unconscious patient the airway is at risk. Regurgitated gastric contents, debris in the mouth or upper airway, loose dentures or mechanical obstruction arising from structures in the mouth, e.g. the tongue and epiglottis, can all compromise the airway (Quinn, 1998).

The recovery position is designed to maintain a patent airway and reduce the risk of airway obstruction and aspiration and is recommended in an unconscious patient who is breathing normally and has an effective circulation (Resuscitation Council (UK), 2012).

NEUROLOGICAL DISORDERS

Indications

The recovery position is advocated for most unconscious patients. In the situation following cardiac arrest, if the patient is breathing spontaneously and does not require any further resuscitation, then appropriate positioning of the patient using the recommended recovery position promotes the maintenance of a clear airway and helps prevent vomit or secretions from obstructing the airway and potentially causing aspiration.

The recovery position is also recommended in many other situations where the patient's conscious level is compromised, e.g. following a major seizure (Hayes, 2004; Bingham, 2004) and during a hypoglycaemic coma (Diebel, 1999).

Right or left lateral

Historically the left lateral position has been advocated for the recovery position (Eastwick-Field, 1996). However, there appears to be no cardiac autonomic tone advantages to be gained by placing a person in the recovery position on one side compared with the other (Ryan *et al.*, 2003). Although either side can be used, in practical terms the environment can dictate which side is used, e.g. if the patient has collapsed next to a wall, he will have to be rolled away from it. In the dental chair, it would be sensible to position the patient so that he is facing the suction apparatus.

Variations

There are several different variations of the recovery position, each with its own advantages (Resuscitation Council (UK), 2011). However, no single technique is perfect for all patients (Turner *et al.*, 1998; Handley, 1993). The position used should be stable, near a true lateral position with the head dependent and no pressure applied to the chest which could impair breathing (American Heart Association, 2005).

Procedure — patient on the floor

- Check the environment and decide which is the best side to roll the patient. Remove any obstacles if necessary.
- If necessary, remove the patient's spectacles and place them in a safe place. Some authorities also recommend checking in the patient's pockets and removing any sharp instruments, e.g. keys. If doing this proceed with extreme caution.
- Loosen any clothing around the neck.

NEUROLOGICAL DISORDERS

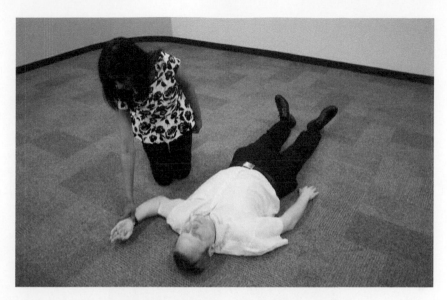

Figure 7.3 Position the arm nearest to the dental practitioner perpendicular to the patient's body with the elbow bent and the hand palm uppermost.

- Kneel beside the patient. To minimise the risk of self-injury, adopt a stable base with the knees a shoulder-width apart, avoid twisting the back and keep the spine in a neutral position (Resuscitation Council (UK), 2009).
- Ensure that both of the patient's legs are straight.
- Position the arm nearest to the dental practitioner perpendicular to the patient's body with the elbow bent and the hand palm uppermost (Figure 7.3).
- Grasp the far arm and bring it across the patient's chest and hold the back of the hand against the patient's cheek.
- Using the free hand, grasp the far leg just above the knee and pull it up, taking care to keep the patient's foot on the ground (Figure 7.4).
- While holding the patient's hand against his cheek, pull on the far leg to roll the patient towards you onto his side.
- Tilt the patient's head back to ensure that the airway remains open (Figure 7.5).
- If necessary, adjust the hand under the patient's cheek to maintain the head tilted.
- Monitor the patient's vital signs.

Source: Resuscitation Council (UK) (2011)

Procedure – patient in the dental chair

Due to limited space, it is very difficult to follow the above procedure when trying to place a patient with altered consciousness in the chair in the recovery position. It will usually be necessary to adapt the procedure. *Note:* there is the

NEUROLOGICAL DISORDERS

NEUROLOGICAL DISORDERS

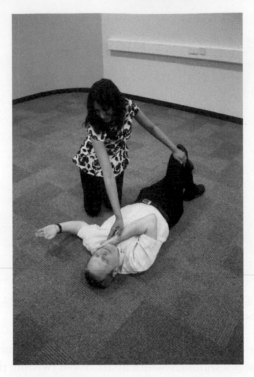

Figure 7.4 The recovery position: grasp the far leg just above the knee and pull it up and roll the patient towards you.

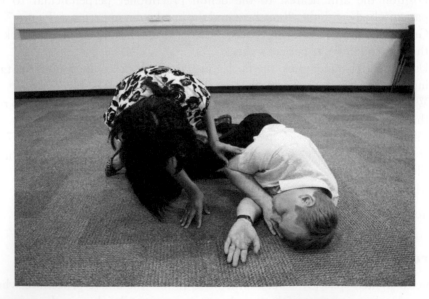

Figure 7.5 The recovery position: tilt the patient's head back to ensure that the airway remains open.

potential hazard of the patient rolling off the chair onto the floor. Great care should be taken when attempting to place the patient in the lateral position in the dental chair.

Safer handling

Guidelines from the Resuscitation Council (UK) (2009) on safer handling during resuscitation should be observed to reduce the risk of self-injury:

- Assess the situation;
- Adopt a position close to and directly facing the patient;
- Avoid twisting the back;
- Keep the spine in a neutral position;
- Face the patient straight on.

Complications

Even if the patient is in the recovery position, airway, breathing and circulation can still become compromised. Closely monitor the patient's vital signs, particularly breathing (Resuscitation Council (UK), 2011).

It has been reported that when the lower arm is placed in front, compression of vessels and nerves in the dependent limb can occur (Fulstow and Smith, 1993; Turner et al., 1998). Therefore monitor for signs of impaired blood flow in the lowermost arm (Rathgeber et al., 1996) and ensure that the duration for which there is pressure on this arm is kept to a minimum (Resuscitation Council (UK), 2011). If the patient needs to remain in the recovery position for longer than 30 minutes, turn him to the opposite side to relieve pressure on the forearm (Resuscitation Council (UK), 2011).

SPINAL INJURY

The author acknowledges that the risk of encountering a spinal injury in the dental practice is extremely rare. However, for completeness, it was considered important to consider it here.

If the patient has a known or suspected spinal injury, he should only be moved if an open airway cannot otherwise be maintained. Ideally the patient should be kept still in the position he is found, while awaiting the arrival of the emergency services. However if it is necessary to move the patient, e.g. because of compromised airway, the patient should ideally be carefully log-rolled, with the head and neck kept as still as possible and in alignment. Extension of the lower arm above the head together with bending both legs, while rolling the head onto the arm, may be feasible (American Heart Association, 2005).

CONCLUSION

Neurological disorders can be life threatening and can occur in the dental practice. An altered consciousness level can lead to a compromised airway and compromised breathing which, if untreated, may lead to cardiopulmonary arrest. The patient should be assessed following the ABCDE approach. In this chapter the management of seizures, stroke and altered level of consciousness have been discussed. In addition, the recovery position, which is often indicated in a patient with a neurological disorder, has been described.

REFERENCES

American Heart Association (2005) 2005 American Heart Association Guidelines for Cardiopulmonary Resuscitation and Emergency cardiovascular care. *Circulation*; 112(24 suppl): IV1–203.

Bassett C, Makin L (eds) (2000) *Caring for the Seriously Ill Patient*. Arnold, London.

Bingham E (2004) Epilepsy: diagnosis and support for people with epilepsy. *Practice Nursing*; 15(2):64–70.

British Medical Association and Royal Pharmaceutical Society of Great Britain (2013) *British National Formulary 65*. BMJ Publishing, London.

Buck D, Baker G, Jacoby A *et al.* (1997) Patients' experiences of injury as a result of epilepsy. *Epilepsia*; 38(4):439–444.

Diebel G (1999) The management of hypoglycaemia in type 1 and type 2 diabetes. *British Journal of Community Nursing*; 4(9):454–460.

Eastwick-Field P (1996) Resuscitation: basic life support. *Nursing Standard*; 10(34):49–56.

Epilepsy Action (2013) www.epilepsy.org.uk (accessed 20 April 2013).

Fulstow R, Smith G (1993) The new recovery position, a cautionary tale. *Resuscitation*; 26:89–91.

Geraghty M (2005) Nursing the unconscious patient. *Nursing Standard*; 20(1):54–64.

Handley A (1993) Recovery position. *Resuscitation*; 26:93–95.

Hayes C (2004) Clinical skills: practical guide for managing adults with epilepsy. *British Journal of Nursing*; 13(7):380–387.

Jevon P (2006) *Emergency Care & First Aid for Nurses*. Elsevier, Oxford.

Jevon P, Morgan A (2007) First aid part 2 – treatment of a generalised tonic-clonic seizure. *Nursing Times*; 103(51):24–25.

Mant J, Walker M (2011) *ABC of Stroke*. Wiley-Blackwell, Oxford.

Müller M, Hänsel M, Stehr S *et al.* (2008) A state-wide survey of medical emergency management in dental practices: incidence of emergencies and training experience. *Emergency Medicine Journal*; 25:296–300.

National Institute for Clinical Excellence (2002) Press Release: 2002/026 NICE launches National Clinical audit of epilepsy-related death, www.nice.org.uk (accessed 20 April 2013).

National Institute for Clinical Excellence (2012) *The Epilepsies: the Diagnosis and Management of the Epilepsies in Adults and Children in Primary and Secondary Care*, http://guidance.nice.org.uk/CG137/NICEGuidance/pdf/English (accessed 1 May 2013).

National Society for Epilepsy (2013) *Epilepsy: What to do When Someone has a Seizure*. National Society for Epilepsy, Chalfont St Peter, Buckinghamshire.

Quinn T (1998) Cardiopulmonary resuscitation: new European guidelines. *British Journal of Nursing*; 7(18):1070–1077.

Rathgeber J, Panzer W, Gunther U *et al*. (1996) Influence of different types of recovery positions on perfusion indices of the forearm. *Resuscitation*; 32:13–17.

Resuscitation Council (UK) (2009) *Guidance for Safer Handling during Resuscitation in Healthcare Settings*. Resuscitation Council (UK), London.

Resuscitation Council (UK) (2011) *Advanced Life Support,* 6th edn. Resuscitation Council (UK), London.

Resuscitation Council (UK) (2012) *Medical Emergencies and Resuscitation Standards for Clinical Practice and Training for Dental Practitioners and Dental Care Professionals in General Dental Practice*. Resuscitation Council (UK), London.

Ryan A, Larsen P, Galletly D (2003) Comparison of heart rate variability in supine, and left and right lateral positions. *Anaesthesia*; 58(5):432–436.

Sharief M, Anand P (1997) Neurological emergencies. In: Skinner D Swain A, Peyton R, *et al*. (eds.) *Cambridge Textbook of Accident & Emergency Medicine*. Cambridge University Press, Cambridge.

St John Ambulance, St Andrew's Ambulance, British Red Cross (2011) *First Aid Manual*, 9th edn. Dorling Kindersley, London.

Scottish Intercollegiate Guidelines Network (2003) *Diagnosis and Management of Epilepsy in Adults*. SIGN, Edinburgh.

Soanes C, Stevenson A (2006) *Oxford Dictionary of English*, 2nd edn. Oxford University Press, Oxford.

The Stroke Association (2013) www.stroke.org.uk (accessed 3 May 2013).

Turner C (2007) *Neurology*, 2nd edn. Mosby, London.

Turner S, Turner I, Chapman D *et al*. (1998) A comparative study of the 1992 and 1997 recovery positions for use in the UK. *Resuscitation*; 39:153–160.

Wyatt J, Illingworth R, Graham C *et al*. (2012) *Oxford Handbook of Emergency Medicine*, 5th edn. Oxford University Press, Oxford.

NEUROLOGICAL DISORDERS

Chapter 8

Anaphylaxis

INTRODUCTION

Anaphylaxis is a life-threatening emergency which can occur in the dental practice (Müller *et al.*, 2008). Anaphylaxis in the dental practice is very rare, accounting for approximately 1% of all encountered emergencies (Müller *et al.*, 2008). It may follow the administration of a drug, e.g. local anaesthetic, or exposure to a substance such as latex (Resuscitation Council (UK), 2012a). In the general population, the incidence of anaphylaxis is on the increase (Department of Health, 2006), probably associated with a notable increase in the prevalence of allergic diseases in the last 30 years (Resuscitation Council (UK), 2012a).

The recent death of a patient, who suffered an anaphylactic reaction and died in a dental practice in Brighton following treatment with corsodyl mouthwash (BBC, 2013), stresses the need for all dental practitioners to be able to recognize and effectively manage anaphylaxis. The Resuscitation Council (UK) (2012a) and NICE (2011) have published guidelines for the management of anaphylaxis.

The aim of this chapter is to understand the emergency management of anaphylaxis.

LEARNING OUTCOMES

At the end of this chapter, the reader will be able to:

- Define anaphylaxis
- Discuss the incidence of anaphylaxis
- Discuss the pathophysiology of anaphylaxis
- List the causes of anaphylaxis
- Describe the clinical features and diagnosis of anaphylaxis
- Discuss the treatment of anaphylaxis

Basic Guide to Medical Emergencies in the Dental Practice, Second Edition. Phil Jevon.
© 2014 John Wiley & Sons, Ltd. Published 2014 by John Wiley & Sons, Ltd.
Companion website: www.wiley.com\go\jevon\medicalemergencies

DEFINITION

Anaphylaxis can be defined as 'a severe, life-threatening, generalised or systemic hypersensitivity reaction' (Johansson *et al.*, 2004). Basically, it is a life-threatening allergic reaction – the extreme end of the allergic spectrum (Anaphylaxis Campaign, 2013).

INCIDENCE

Available UK estimates suggest that approximately 1 in 1300 of the population of England has experienced anaphylaxis at some point in their lives (NICE, 2011). There has also been a dramatic rise in the rate of hospital admissions for anaphylaxis. Between 1990 and 2004 they increased from 0.5 admissions per 100,000 to 3.6 per 100,000, an increase of 700% (Gupta *et al.*, 2007), and there are now around 20 deaths each year in the United Kingdom from anaphylaxis (although this may be a substantial underestimate) (NICE, 2011). In a survey of 620 dental surgeries, 7 had encountered anaphylaxis in the previous 12 month period (Müller *et al.*, 2008).

Anaphylaxis is more common in females than in males. In 2004, 58% of attendees to emergency departments with anaphylaxis were female, 42% were male (Peng and Jick, 2004); Webb and Lieberman's (2006) findings were comparable: 62% females and 38% males. The mean age of patient with anaphylaxis is 37 years (Webb and Lieberman, 2006).

From the author's experience (feedback from dental practitioners), cases of anaphylaxis in the dental practice have been caused by a number of factors including local anaesthetic, latex, amoxycillin and metronidazole.

PATHOPHYSIOLOGY

Irrespective of the mechanism of anaphylaxis, mast cells and basophils release histamines and other vasoactive mediators which produce circulatory, respiratory, gastrointestinal and cutaneous effects (Wyatt *et al.*, 2012). These effects can include the development of pharyngeal and laryngeal oedema, bronchospasm, decreased vascular tone and capillary leak causing circulatory collapse (Jevon, 2004).

ANAPHYLAXIS

CAUSES

Causes of anaphylaxis include:

- drugs, e.g. penicillin, aspirin, local anaesthetic, surface anaesthetics (e.g. benzocaine);
- bee/wasp stings;
- foods, e.g. peanuts, tomatoes, fish;
- latex.

Source: British Medical Association and Royal Pharmaceutical Society (2013), Jevon (2008), Anaphylaxis Campaign (2013)

    Table 8.1 lists suspected triggers for fatal anaphylactic reactions in the United Kingdom between 1992 and 2001 (Pumphrey, 2004). When anaphylaxis is fatal, death usually occurs very soon following contact with the trigger (Resuscitation Council (UK), 2012a). In fatal food anaphylactic reactions, respiratory arrest usually occurs after 30–35 minutes; in fatal

Table 8.1 Suspected triggers for fatal anaphylactic reactions in the United Kingdom between 1992 and 2001

Cause	Number of cases	Breakdown
Stings	47	29 Wasp, 4 bee, 14 unknown
Nuts	32	10 Peanut, 6 walnut, 2 almond, 2 Brazil, 1 hazel, 11 mixed or unknown
Food	13	5 Milk, 2 chickpea, 2 crustacean, 1 banana, 1 snail
Food possible cause	17	5 During meal, 3 milk, 3 nut, 1 each – fish, yeast, sherbet, nectarine, grape, strawberry
Antibiotics	27	11 Penicillin, 12 Cephalosporin, 2 Amphotericin, 1 Ciprofloxacin, 1 Vancomycin
Anaesthetic drugs	39	19 Suxamethonium, 7 Vecuronium, 6 Atracurium, 7 At Induction
Other drugs	24	6 NSAID, 3 ACEI, 5 Gelatins, 2 protamine, 2 vitamin K, 1 each – etoposide, Acetazolamide, Pethidine, local anaesthetic, Diamorphine, Streptokinase
Contrast media	11	9 Iodinated, 1 Technetium, 1 Fluorescein
Other	3	1 Latex, 1 Hair Dye, 1 Hydatid (tape worm cyst)

Sources: Pumphrey (2004) and Resuscitation Council (UK) (2012a).

insect sting anaphylactic reactions, cardiovascular shock usually occurs after 10–15 minutes; and in fatal intravenous medication anaphylactic reactions, cardiac arrest occurs most commonly within 5 minutes (Pumphrey, 2000). Death never occurred more than 6 hours after contact with the trigger (Pumphrey, 2000).

Anaphylaxis can also be associated with additives and excipients (an excipient is an inactive substance that serves as a vehicle or medium for a drug (Soanes and Stevenson, 2006)). It is therefore recommended to check the full formula of preparations, including those for topical application, especially those intended for use in the mouth (British Medical Association and Royal Pharmaceutical Society, 2013).

In approximately 40% of anaphylactic reactions, the cause is unknown (idiopathic anaphylaxis) (Webb and Lieberman, 2006; Greenberger, 2007).

Local anaesthetic

Following the administration of a local anaesthetic, a minority of patients may suffer one of a range of unwanted symptoms. Some of these symptoms can be mistaken for hypersensitivity or allergy and the patient unnecessarily told they are allergic to the anaesthetic (Henderson, 2011). Allergy to local anaesthetic is rare (more likely with the ester local anaesthetic agents – not used routinely in dentistry) (Henderson, 2011). Due to the rarity of local anaesthetic allergy, if a patient experiences signs and symptoms suggestive of an allergic response, it is prudent to consider other possible causes of the symptoms, e.g. toxicity (sedation, light headedness, slurred speech, mood alteration, diplopia, disorientation and muscle twitching) (Henderson, 2011).

ANAPHYLAXIS

CLINICAL FEATURES AND DIAGNOSIS

The lack of a consistent clinical picture can sometimes make an accurate diagnosis difficult (Project Team of the Resuscitation Council (UK), 2012a). Anaphylaxis can vary in severity and the process can be slow, rapid or biphasic; occasionally the onset may be delayed by a few hours and even persist for longer than 24 hours (Fisher, 1986). As soon as possible a detailed history should be taken and the patient should be examined. The clinical presentation often includes:

- Urticaria (Figure 8.1) (a rash of round, red weals on the skin which itch intensely; sometimes referred to as nettle rash or hives), erythema, rhinitis, conjunctivitis;
- Flushing – common, but pallor may also occur;

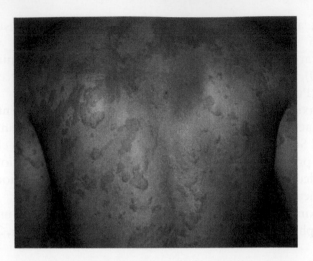

Figure 8.1 Urticaria. *Source:* From Dr J. Halpern, Consultant Dermatologist.

- Angioedema (Figure 8.2);
- Marked upper airway (laryngeal) oedema and bronchospasm – causing stridor, wheezing and/or a hoarse voice;
- Vasodilation causing hypovolemia leading to low blood pressure and collapse. This can cause cardiac arrest;
- Abdominal pain, vomiting, diarrhoea and a sense of impending doom.

Source: Jevon (2008), Anaphylaxis Campaign (2013)

Anaphylaxis can vary in severity and the onset is usually rapid; occasionally it may be delayed by a few hours and may even persist for longer than 24 hours (Fisher, 1986). The patient feels unwell, usually has skin changes, e.g. urticaria, and angioedema and will have a compromised airway and/or

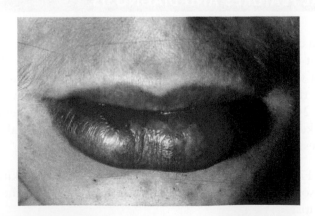

Figure 8.2 Angioedema. *Source:* From Dr J. Halpern, Consultant Dermatologist.

breathing and/or circulation (Jevon, 2008). Death from anaphylaxis usually occurs within 10–15 minutes, with cardiovascular collapse the commonest cause of death (Resuscitation Council (UK), 2012a).

It is possible to mistake a panic attack or a vasovagal attack for anaphylaxis and adrenaline has been administered inappropriately in these situations (Johnston *et al.*, 2003). The clinical features of these presentations (Jevon, 2008) include:

- *Panic attack:* hyperventilation, tachycardia and anxiety-related erythematous (red) rash, but no hypotension, pallor, wheeze or urticarial rash;
- *Vasovagal attack:* relating to or denoting a temporary fall in blood pressure, with pallor, collapse, sweating and nausea, caused by overactivity of the vagus nerve particularly as a result of stress (Soanes and Stevenson, 2006): the absence of a rash, tachycardia and dyspnoea should rule out anaphylaxis as the cause of the collapse.

TREATMENT

The Resuscitation Council (UK) algorithm for the treatment of anaphylaxis in adults in the community is detailed in Figure 8.3. The treatment of anaphylaxis is as follows (Resuscitation Council (UK), 2012b):

- Assess the patient following the ABCDE approach described in Chapter 3.
- Call for help from colleagues and call 999 for an ambulance. Request adrenaline as well as emergency equipment including oxygen.
- If able, stop or remove the probable cause of the anaphylaxis, e.g. remove latex gloves.
- Ensure the patient is in a comfortable position: patients with airway and breathing difficulties may prefer to sit up while those with hypotension usually befit from lying down with the legs raised.
- Administer 15 l of oxygen through a non-rebreather oxygen mask (see Figure 3.1); if available, establish oxygen saturation monitoring using a pulse oximeter.
- For severe reactions where there are life-threatening airway and/or breathing and/or circulation problems, i.e., hoarseness, stridor, severe wheeze, cyanosis, pale, clammy, drowsy, confusion or coma: administer adrenaline 500 µg (0.5 ml of 1:1000 solution) IM.
- Repeat the adrenaline after 5 minutes if there is no improvement (further doses of adrenaline at 5 minute intervals may be required).
- Do not sit the patient up or stand him up if he is feeling faint or dizzy – he may be in profound shock and may then have a cardiac arrest.
- When able to do so, record the circumstances immediately before the onset of symptoms to help to identify the possible trigger of the anaphylactic

ANAPHYLAXIS

Anaphylactic reactions – Initial treatment

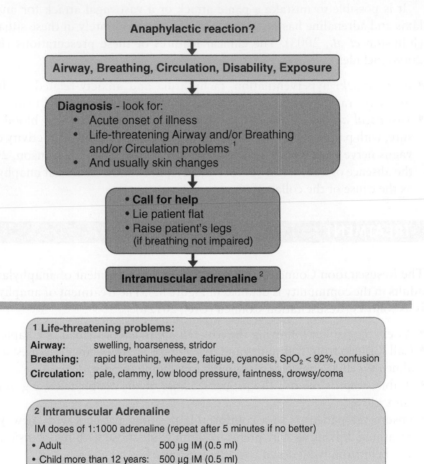

Anaphylactic reaction?

↓

Airway, Breathing, Circulation, Disability, Exposure

↓

Diagnosis - look for:
- Acute onset of illness
- Life-threatening Airway and/or Breathing and/or Circulation problems [1]
- And usually skin changes

↓

- **Call for help**
- Lie patient flat
- Raise patient's legs
  (if breathing not impaired)

↓

Intramuscular adrenaline [2]

[1] Life-threatening problems:

Airway: swelling, hoarseness, stridor
Breathing: rapid breathing, wheeze, fatigue, cyanosis, SpO_2 < 92%, confusion
Circulation: pale, clammy, low blood pressure, faintness, drowsy/coma

[2] Intramuscular Adrenaline

IM doses of 1:1000 adrenaline (repeat after 5 minutes if no better)

- Adult   500 µg IM (0.5 ml)
- Child more than 12 years: 500 µg IM (0.5 ml)
- Child 6–12 years: 300 µg IM (0.3 ml)
- Child less than 6 years: 150 µg IM (0.15 ml)

Figure 8.3 Resuscitation Council (UK) algorithm for the management of anaphylaxis. *Source:* Resuscitation Council (UK). Reproduced with permission.

reaction, the acute clinical features of the suspected anaphylactic reaction and the time of onset of the reaction.

In the event of anaphylaxis, do not delay giving adrenaline if available. Adrenaline is the first treatment of anaphylaxis, even before oxygen and other resuscitation steps (Allergy UK, 2013)

Adrenaline

Adrenaline (Figure 8.4) is the most important drug in anaphylaxis (Fisher, 1995). To be effective, it needs to be administered promptly (Patel *et al.*, 1994). Adrenaline:

- reverses peripheral vasodilation;
- reduces oedema;
- dilates the airways;
- increases myocardial contractility;
- suppresses histamine and leukotriene release.

The recommended dose of adrenaline is 500 µg (0.5 ml of 1:1000 solution) intramuscularly (thigh) (British Medical Association and Royal Pharmaceutical Society, 2013). This can be repeated after 5 minutes if there is no clinical improvement (Resuscitation Council (UK), 2012a); several doses may be required (British Medical Association and Royal Pharmaceutical Society, 2013). The intramuscular route for the administration of adrenaline should be used as it is relatively safe and adverse effects are rare. The only reported severe adverse effect following intramuscular administration of adrenaline was a myocardial infarction in a patient with severe ischaemic heart disease (Saff *et al.*, 1993).

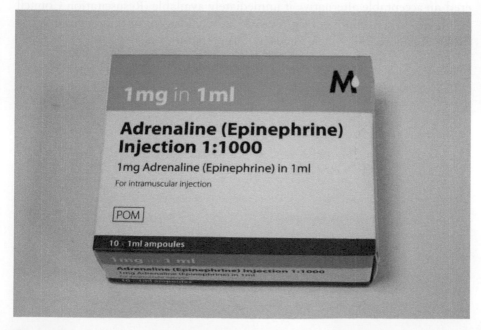

Figure 8.4 Adrenaline 1:1000 solution (1 mg in 1 ml).

ANAPHYLAXIS

When using adrenaline 1:1000 ampoules, it is recommended to use a 23 g (blue), or in a larger patient, a 21 g (green) needle, to draw up and administer the required dose. Dental practitioners will probably find an adrenaline 1:1000 prefilled syringe (Figure 8.5) (i.e. not having to draw up the drug from an ampoule) helpful. Care should be taken to ensure that the correct dose is administered.

Paediatric doses of adrenaline:

- 6–12 years of age – 300 μg IM (0.3 ml of 1:1000 adrenaline)
- 6 years – 150 μg IM (0.15 ml of 1:1000 adrenaline)

Cautions include the following:

- Two strengths of adrenaline are available: 1:1000 solution is used for intramuscular injection, while the 1:10,000 solution that some dental practices stock, is used for intravenous injection during cardiopulmonary resuscitation (Jevon, 2008).
- The subcutaneous route for the administration of adrenaline should not be utilised because absorption is considerably slower (Simons *et al.*, 1998).

Adrenaline auto-injector device

If the patient has an adrenaline auto-injector device (Figure 8.6), this is considered an acceptable alternative if immediately available (Resuscitation Council (UK), 2012a). A commonly prescribed adrenaline self-injector device is the EPIPEN (Figure 8.6) which comes in two preparations.

- 300 μg single dose: for adults and children over 30 kg (aged approximately 11+ years).

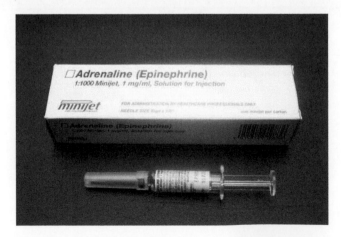

Figure 8.5 Adrenaline 1:1000 pre-filled syringe.

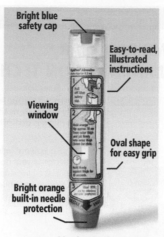

Bright blue
safety cap

Easy-to-read,
illustrated
instructions

Viewing
window

Oval shape
for easy grip

Bright orange
built-in needle
protection

Comes with a free hard carry case

Figure 8.6 EpiPen. *Source:* Meda. Reproduced with permission.

- 150 µg single dose: for children 15–30 kg (aged approximately 4–11 years) (British Medical Association and Royal Pharmaceutical Society, 2013).

  Guidelines for using an EpiPen are given in Box 8.1.

> There is no legal problem in any person administering adrenaline for treatment of a possible anaphylactic reaction (Allergy UK, 2013)

Inhaled beta-2 agonist

Consider further bronchodilatory therapy, e.g. salbutamol inhaler (Resuscitation Council (UK), 2012a).

Reporting of reaction

Adverse drug reactions that include anaphylaxis should be reported to the Medicines and Healthcare products Regulatory Agency (MHRA) using the yellow card scheme (www.mhra.gov.uk). Copies of the yellow card can be found in the back of The British National Formulary (BNF).

RISK ASSESSMENT

A medical and drug history will enable the Dental Practitioner to identify if a patient is at a particular risk of having an anaphylactic reaction and can then take measures to reduce the chance of a problem arising (Resuscitation Council

Box 8.1   Procedure for using an EpiPen

SAME FAMILIAR
ADMINISTRATION TECHNIQUE

Step 1 — Lie down with your legs slightly elevated or sit up if breathing is difficult

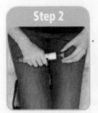

Step 2 — Grasp your **EpiPen®**(adrenaline) auto-injector in your dominant hand with the blue safety cap closest to your thumb and remove cap

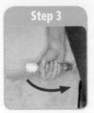

Step 3 — Hold your **EpiPen®**(adrenaline) auto-injector about 10 cm away from your leg and **swing and jab** the orange tip into the upper outer thigh at a 90° angle

Hold in place for 10 seconds

Remove the **EpiPen®**(adrenaline) auto-injector and massage injection site for at least 10 seconds

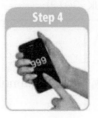

Step 4 — **You must dial 999**, ask for an ambulance and **state 'anaphylaxis'** (pronounced 'anna-fill-axis') immediately after administering the **EpiPen®**(adrenaline) auto-injector

Do not get up, stay lying down or seated until you have been assessed by a paramedic

Source: Meda. Reproduced with permission.

(UK), 2012a), e.g. if the patient is known to have a latex allergy, ensure that latex-free gloves are used.

CONCLUSION

Anaphylaxis can be life threatening. This chapter has detailed the guidelines issued by the Resuscitation Council (UK) to treat it (Resuscitation Council (UK), 2012a). Early treatment with intramuscular adrenaline is paramount.

REFERENCES

Allergy UK (2013) www.allergyuk.org (accessed 05 May 2013).

Anaphylaxis Campaign (2013) www.anaphylaxis.org.uk (accessed 05 May 2013).

BBC *Mouthwash reaction killed Brighton dental patient,* http://www.bbc.co.uk/news/uk-england-sussex-14951073 (accessed 4 January 2013).

British Medical Association and Royal Pharmaceutical Society of Great Britain (2013) *BNF 65.* BMJ Publishing, London.

Department of Health (2006) *A Review of Services for Allergy: The Epidemiology, Demand for, and Provision of Treatment and Effectiveness of Clinical Interventions.* Department of Health, London.

Fisher M (1986) Clinical observations on the pathophysiology and treatment of anaphylactic cardiovascular collapse. *Anaesthesia and Intensive Care*; 14:17–21.

Fisher M (1995) Treatment of acute anaphylaxis. *BMJ*; 311:731–733.

Greenberger P (2007) Idiopathic anaphylaxis. *Immunology and Allergy Clinics of North America*; 27(2):273–293.

Gupta R, Sheikh A, Strachan D, Anderson H (2007) Time trends in allergic disorders in the UK. *Thorax*; 62:91–96.

Henderson S (2011) Allergy to local anaesthetic agents used in dentistry—what are the signs, symptoms, alternative diagnoses and management options? *Dental Update*; 38(6):410–412.

Jevon P (2004) *Anaphylaxis: A Practical Guide.* Butterworth Heinemann, Oxford.

Jevon P (2008) Severe allergic reaction: management of anaphylaxis in hospital. *British Journal of Nursing*; 17(2):104–108.

Johansson S, Bieber T, Dhal R *et al.* (2004) Revised nomenclature for allergy for global use: report of the Nomenclature Review Committee of the World Allergy Organization, October 2003. *Journal of Allergy and Clinical Immunology*; 113(5):832–836.

Johnston S, Unsworth J, Gompels M (2003) Adrenaline given outside the context of life-threatening allergic reactions. *BMJ*; 326(7389):589–590.

Müller M, Hänsel M, Stehr S *et al.* (2008) A state-wide survey of medical emergency management in dental practices: incidence of emergencies and training experience. *Emergency Medicine Journal*; 25:296–300.

NICE (2011) *Guideline CG134 Initial assessment and referral following emergency treatment for an anaphylactic episode.* www.nice.org.uk (accessed 04 October 2013).

Patel L, Radivan FS, David TJ (1994) Management of anaphylactic reactions to food. *Archives of Disease in Childhood*; 71:370–375.

Peng M, Jick H (2004) A population-based study of the incidence, cause and severity of anaphylaxis in the United Kingdom. *Archives of Internal Medicine*; 164(3):317–319.

Pumphrey RSH (2000) Lessons for management of anaphylaxis from a study of fatal reactions. *Clinical and Experimental Allergy*; 30(8):1144–1150.

Pumphrey RSH (2004) Fatal anaphylaxis in the UK, 1992–2001. *Novartis Foundation Symposium*; 257:116–128; discussion 128–132, 157–160, 276–285.

Resuscitation Council (UK) (2012a) *Emergency Medical Treatment of Anaphylactic Reactions.* Resuscitation Council (UK), London.

Resuscitation Council (UK) (2012b) *Medical Emergencies and Resuscitation Standards for Clinical Practice and Training for Dental Practitioners and Dental Care Professionals in General Dental Practice.* Resuscitation Council (UK), London.

ANAPHYLAXIS

Saff R, Nahhas A, Fink J (1993) Myocardial infarction induced by coronary vasospasm after self-administration of epinephrine. *Annals of Allergy*; 70:396–398.

Simons F, Roberts J, Gu X, Simons K (1998) Epinephrine absorption in children with a history of anaphylaxis. *Journal of Allergy and Clinical Immunology*; 101:33–37.

Soanes C, Stevenson A (2006) *Oxford Dictionary of English*, 2nd edn. Oxford University Press, Oxford.

Webb L, Lieberman P (2006) Anaphylaxis: a review of 601 cases. *Annals of Allergy, Asthma & Immunology*; 97(1):39–43.

Wyatt J, Illingworth R, Graham C *et al.* (2012) *Oxford Handbook of Emergency Medicine*, 4th edn. Oxford University Press, Oxford.

ANAPHYLAXIS

Chapter 9

Cardiopulmonary resuscitation in the dental practice

INTRODUCTION

Cardiopulmonary arrest accounts for 0.3% of all medical emergencies encountered in the dental practice (Müller *et al.*, 2008). A recent study showed that cardiopulmonary arrest occurs in 1 in approximately 300,000 patients (Müller *et al.*, 2008).

Effective cardiopulmonary resuscitation (CPR) and early defibrillation are the only two interventions that have been shown to improve survival following a cardiopulmonary arrest: attention must therefore be focused on these while undertaking CPR. Following guidance from the Resuscitation Council (UK) (2012), dental practices are purchasing automated external defibrillators (AEDs), thus enabling defibrillation before the arrival of the ambulance (if indicated). The procedure for using an AED is discussed in detail in Chapter 11. The principles of airway management and ventilation are discussed in detail in Chapter 10.

The aim of this chapter is to understand the procedure for CPR in the dental practice.

LEARNING OUTCOMES

At the end of the chapter, the reader will be able to:

- Discuss the background to the Resuscitation Council (UK) automated external defibrillation algorithm
- Outline the procedure for CPR in the chair
- Discuss the principles of chest compressions

Basic Guide to Medical Emergencies in the Dental Practice, Second Edition. Phil Jevon.
© 2014 John Wiley & Sons, Ltd. Published 2014 by John Wiley & Sons, Ltd.
Companion website: www.wiley.com\go\jevon\medicalemergencies

RESUSCITATION COUNCIL (UK) AUTOMATED EXTERNAL DEFIBRILLATION ALGORITHM

Ventricular fibrillation (see Chapter 1) is the commonest primary arrhythmia at the onset of an adult cardiac arrest outside hospital (Resuscitation Council (UK), 2011).

It is an eminently treatable rhythm, with most eventual survivors coming from this group (Tunstall-Pedoe et al., 1992). Early defibrillation is the definitive treatment; the chances of success decline substantially with each passing minute. This process can be slowed, but not halted, by effective basic life support (Resuscitation Council (UK), 2011). Effective CPR and prompt defibrillation within the first few minutes of the onset of cardiac arrest can produce survival rates as high as 75% (Colquhoun et al., 2008).

The Resuscitation Council (UK) automated external defibrillation algorithm (Figure 9.1) therefore focuses on the need to minimise any delay between the onset of cardiac arrest and defibrillation, if it is required. Until an AED is attached, only the first part of the algorithm will be followed (up to CPR 30:2). Hopefully, the dental practice will have immediate access to an AED, thus facilitating its early attachment and, if indicated, rapid defibrillation. Otherwise, CPR 30:2 will need to be performed while awaiting the emergency ambulance.

Modern AEDs will be programmed to follow the current Resuscitation Council (UK) automated external defibrillation algorithm (Resuscitation Council (UK), 2012). Some older AEDs may follow previous (pre-December 2005) guidelines. Some of these devices can be simply updated in line with the current guidelines (usually with an inexpensive item of software); others will not. If the latter is the case, the user should follow the AED's instructions (Resuscitation Council (UK), 2006).

The automated external defibrillation algorithm is designed to be an aide-memoire, reminding the practitioner of the important aspects of assessment and treatment of cardiac arrest. It is not designed to be comprehensive or limiting. Each step that follows in the algorithm assumes that the previous one has been unsuccessful. Looping the algorithm reinforces the concept of constant assessment and reassessment.

PROCEDURE FOR CARDIOPULMONARY RESUSCITATION IN THE DENTAL CHAIR

The procedures described below and the sequences in which the actions are carried out are based on Resuscitation Council (UK) (2011) recommendations and the automated external defibrillation algorithm. When more than one dental practitioner is present some of the actions described will be undertaken

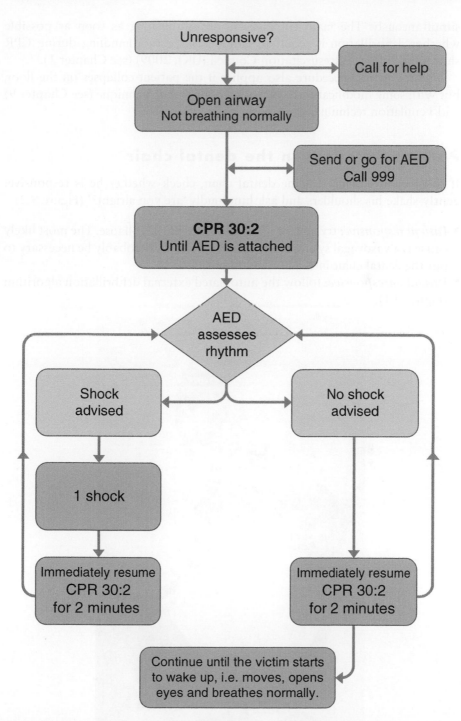

Figure 9.1 Resuscitation Council (UK) automated external defibrillation algorithm.
Source: Resuscitation Council (UK). Reproduced with permission.

simultaneously. The main emphasis is on establishing as soon as possible whether defibrillation is required. Guidelines for safe handling during CPR should be followed (Resuscitation Council (UK), 2009) (see Chapter 1).

The following procedure also applies if the patient collapses on the floor, but with some modifications, e.g. chest compression technique (see Chapter 9) and ventilation technique (see Chapter 10).

Patient collapses in the dental chair

If the patient collapses in the dental chair, check whether he is responsive: gently shake his shoulders and ask him loudly 'are you alright?' (Figure 9.2).

- *Patient responsive:* try and establish the cause of the collapse. The most likely cause is a vasovagal syncope (see Chapter 7). It will probably be necessary to put the dental chair into a horizontal position.
- *Patient unresponsive:* follow the automated external defibrillation algorithm (Figure 9.1).

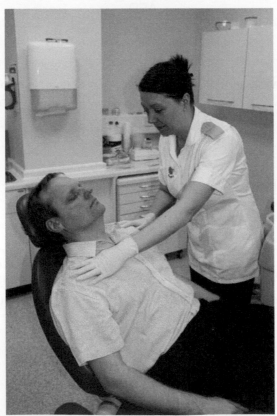

Figure 9.2 CPR: assess responsiveness – gently shake and shout.

Unresponsive

- Call for help from colleagues following local protocol. For example, this may simply involve shouting 'help' or shouting a certain code word such as 'code red', pressing an emergency buzzer or sending a message via the computer system. It would be helpful if a colleague could fetch the emergency equipment and oxygen.
- If not already done, recline the dental chair into the horizontal position. It is possible on most dental chairs to press an emergency button on the chair to activate this position.

Open airway

As the patient is unresponsive and appears to be lifeless, it is important to establish whether he has had a cardiopulmonary arrest. Open the airway and look for signs of life.

- Open the airway by tilting the head and lifting the chin.
- Ensure the airway is clear; it may be necessary to apply suction.
- While maintaining the head tilt and chin lift, assess for signs of normal breathing; look for chest movement (breathing or coughing), listen for breath sounds at the patient's mouth and feel for air on your cheek (Resuscitation Council (UK), 2011) (Figure 9.3). During the first few minutes following a cardiac arrest the patient may be barely breathing and may be taking infrequent noisy gasps; do not mistake this for normal breathing signs of

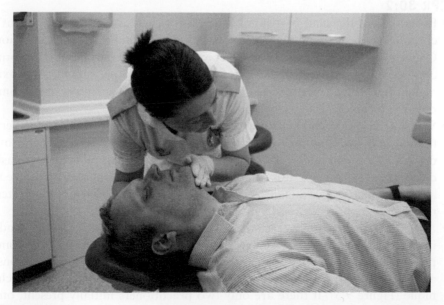

Figure 9.3 CPR: assess for signs of normal breathing – look, listen and feel.

life and circulation (Handley and Colquhoun, 2010; Handley *et al.*, 2010) Also look for movement and other signs of life (Resuscitation Council (UK), 2011). Take no longer than 10 seconds to check for signs of normal breathing (Jevon, 2009).

> Agonal breathing (occasional gasps, slow, laboured or noisy breathing) is common in the early stages of cardiac arrest and is a sign of cardiac arrest and should not be confused as a sign of life/circulation (Resuscitation Council (UK), 2011)

Patient breathing normally

If necessary, request assistance from senior colleagues; assess the patient following the ABCDE approach; administer oxygen if necessary (see Chapter 3). An unresponsive patient who is breathing normally should usually be placed in the lateral position.

Not breathing normally

- Call 999 for an ambulance. Ideally a colleague should be doing this. It would be helpful if a member of the team (if numbers allow) could wait outside the dental practice looking out for the ambulance (a patient may be willing to do this).
- Send or fetch for AED. Ideally, colleagues should bring the AED and resuscitation equipment, while chest compressions are immediately started.

CPR 30:2

- Ensuring that the chair is at suitable height for chest compressions; patient's chest should be between the practitioner's knee and mid-thigh (Resuscitation Council (UK), 2009). Start CPR, 30 compressions to 2 ventilations. Perform chest compressions (Figure 9.4) at a rate of 100–120 per minute (approximately two chest compressions per second). Safe and effective chest compression technique is described below.
- While performing chest compressions, ask colleagues to prepare for ventilation, e.g. inserting an oropharyngeal airway, and connecting high flow oxygen to the ventilatory device, e.g. pocket mask or self-inflating bag-mask device (see Chapter 10). It is important to ensure that a ventilatory device is always immediately available as healthcare personnel should not be expected to perform mouth-to-mouth ventilation.
- After 30 compressions, release the pressure on the chest but leave the hands in situ, while the colleagues deliver two ventilations. Then restart chest compressions. Most dental practices have a self-inflating bag for ventilations: attach oxygen 10 l/min as soon as possible and follow the two-person technique (Figure 9.5). If there are only two practitioners initially present, one could perform chest compressions and then squeeze the bag, while the other

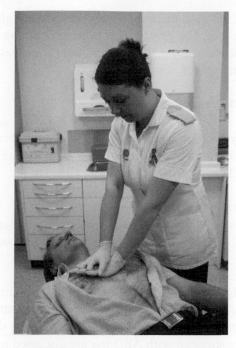

Figure 9.4 CPR: chest compressions.

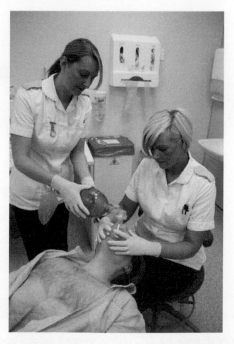

Figure 9.5 CPR: two-person technique for ventilating using a self-inflating bag.

holds the mask on and maintains an open airway (alternatively a pocket mask could be used). The practitioner holding the mask on should ideally be sitting on the dentist's stool. The techniques for airway and ventilation are described in detail in the next chapter.

Until AED is attached

- Once the AED arrives, position it near the patient (e.g. on his lap), switch it on and apply large adhesive electrodes as instructed by the AED; CPR should ideally continue while this is being done (Figure 9.6). The procedure for using an AED is described in detail in Chapter 11.

AED assesses rhythm

- Once the AED starts to assess the rhythm (ECG), ask colleagues to momentarily stop CPR as movement may interfere with this assessment.

Shock advised

- If a shock is advised, the AED will charge up automatically. Ask colleagues to stand clear of the patient and the dental chair and move oxygen at least 1 m away. Perform a quick visual check before pressing the shock button (the safety features associated with AED use are discussed in Chapter 11).

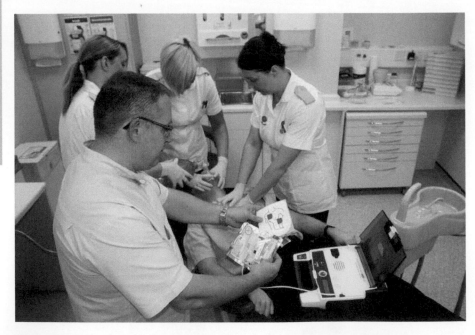

Figure 9.6 Using the AED: once the AED arrives, switch it on and apply large adhesive electrodes.

CARDIOPULMONARY RESUSCITATION IN THE DENTAL PRACTICE

1 shock
- Deliver shock (usually involves pressing a flashing shock button (Figure 9.7), though some AEDs are fully automatic and do not require the operator to do this). The AED will automatically select the shock energy required.

Immediately resume CPR 30:2 for 2 minutes
- Immediately resume chest compressions 30:2 for 2 minutes (Figure 9.8). Only stop CPR if the patient starts to breathe normally or if the AED instructs you to because it is reassessing the ECG.

No shock advised
- Immediately resume chest compressions 30:2 for 2 minutes. Only stop CPR if the patient starts to wake up: to move, opens eyes and to breathe normally or if the AED instructs you to because it is reassessing the ECG.

Continue until the victim starts to wake up: to move, opens eyes and to breathe normally
- While looping the algorithm following the AED's instructions, if the patient starts to wake up (to move, opens eyes and to breathe normally), stop CPR and reassess following the ABCDE approach described in Chapter 3.
- Administer 15 l/min oxygen using a non-rebreathe mask (see Chapter 3).

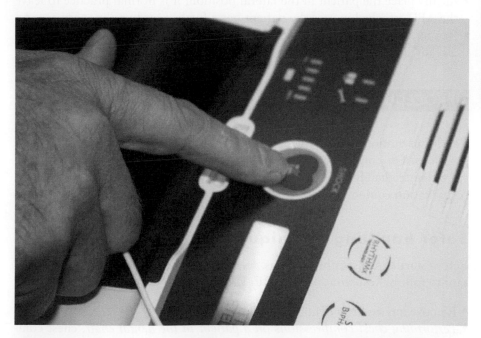

Figure 9.7 Using the AED: deliver shock (usually involves pressing a flashing shock button).

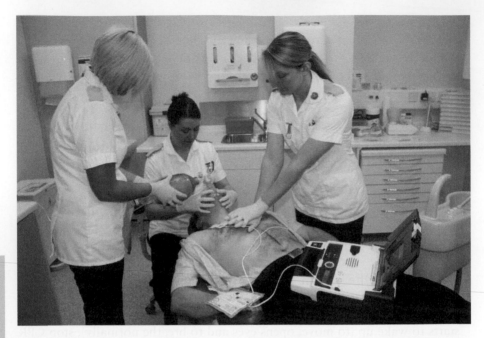

Figure 9.8 Using the AED: after delivery of the shock, restart chest compressions immediately as instructed by the AED. Ideally change over the person performing chest compressions.

- Ideally place the patient in the lateral position; it is normal practice to leave the AED attached in case the patient has a further cardiopulmonary arrest.
- Reassure the patient and ensure that next-of-kin has been informed (if not already done).

PROCEDURE FOR PERFORMING CHEST COMPRESSIONS

The Resuscitation Council (UK) (2011) stresses the importance of chest compressions. On confirmation of cardiac arrest, chest compressions should be started immediately while colleagues call the emergency services and fetch the resuscitation equipment and AED.

Safer handling techniques

Before starting chest compressions, to minimise the risk of injury it is important to follow Resuscitation Council (UK) (2009) safer handling guidelines.

- Remove any environmental hazards.
- *Performing chest compressions on a patient in the dental chair:* chest compressions can be performed effectively in the dental chair (Yokoyama *et al.*,

2008), as long as the correct procedures are followed: ensure the chair is at a height which places the patient between the knee and mid-thigh of the person performing chest compressions; stand at the side of the chair with the feet shoulder-width apart, position the shoulders directly over the patient's sternum and keep the arms straight (Figure 9.9).

- *Performing chest compressions on a patient on the floor:* kneel in the high-kneeling position, at the side of the patient, level with his chest with the knees a shoulder-width apart; position the shoulders directly over the patient's sternum and keep the arms straight (Figure 9.10).

Technique

Once the correct position has been adopted (see Safer handling techniques):

- Place one hand on the centre of the patient's chest (this equates to the middle of the lower half of the sternum) and then place the other on top (this is quicker than spending time on the 'rib margin' location method); do not apply pressure over the end of the sternum or the upper abdomen (Handley and Colquhoun, 2010).

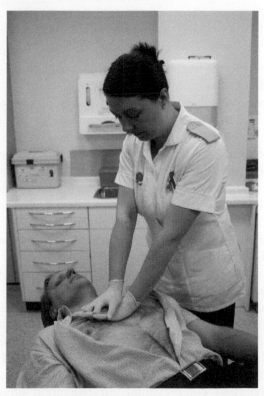

Figure 9.9 Chest compressions in the dental chair.

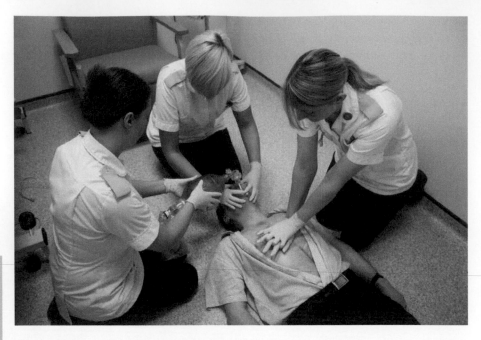

Figure 9.10 Chest compression on the floor.

- Interlock and extend the fingers to avoid applying pressure over the patient's ribs (Figure 9.11).
- Apply pressure to the sternum only; do not apply pressure to the ribs, the end of the sternum or the upper abdomen (Handley and Colquhoun, 2010).
- Position the shoulders directly vertical above the patient's sternum, straighten the arms and lock the elbows; ensure the back is not twisted.
- Compress the sternum 5–6 cm and, following each compression, allow the chest to completely recoil back to its normal position (Handley and Colquhoun, 2010), thus facilitating venous return.
- Ensure that the force of compression results from flexing the hips (Resuscitation Council (UK), 2009).
- Perform chest compressions in a controlled manner; they should not be erratic or jerky.
- Continue chest compressions at a rate of 100–120/min (Handley and Colquhoun, 2010); this rate refers to the speed of compressions rather than the actual number delivered per minute; interruptions in chest compressions, e.g. to allow defibrillation, will result in fewer than 100–120 compressions being delivered in a minute.
- Ensure that the chest compression/chest relaxation phases are of equal duration.

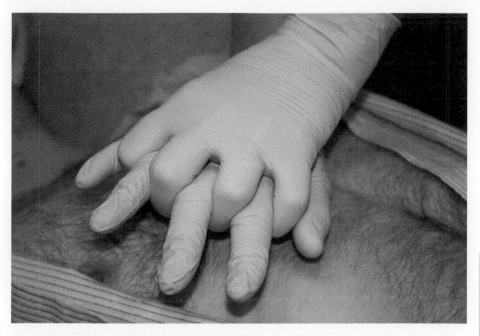

Figure 9.11 Chest compressions: interlock the fingers.

- Ensure a ratio of 30 compressions:2 ventilations (30:2) to allow more time for chest compressions. However, if the airway has been secured, e.g. with a tracheal tube (by the paramedic) asynchronous compressions and ventilations should be performed as this will result in a higher mean coronary perfusion pressure (a pause in chest compressions leads to a substantial fall in this pressure) (Resuscitation Council (UK), 2011).
- To prevent fatigue, rotate the person performing chest compressions approximately every 2 minutes (Resuscitation Council (UK), 2011).

It is important to follow Resuscitation Council (UK)'s (2009) safer handling guidelines during CPR. Ventilate using available airway and ventilation devices. Once the defibrillator arrives, apply ECG leads/defibrillation.

CONCLUSION

Cardiopulmonary arrest in the dental practice is rare. If it does occur, it is important to follow Resuscitation Council (UK) guidelines (2011). In this chapter the Resuscitation Council (UK) automated external defibrillation algorithm has been outlined. The procedure for CPR in the chair and the principles of chest compressions have been discussed.

CARDIOPULMONARY RESUSCITATION
IN THE DENTAL PRACTICE

REFERENCES

Colquhoun MC, Chamberlain DA, Newcombe RG, *et al.* (2008) A national scheme for public access defibrillation in England and Wales: early results. *Resuscitation*; 78:275–80.

Handley A, Colquhoun M (2010) *Adult Basic Life Support,* www.resus.org.uk (accessed 04 May 2013).

Jevon P (2009) *Advanced Cardiac Life Support,* 2nd edn. Wiley-Blackwell, Oxford.

Müller M, Hänsel M, Stehr S *et al.* (2008) A state-wide survey of medical emergency management in dental practices: incidence of emergencies and training experience. *Emergency Medicine Journal*; 25:296–300.

Resuscitation Council (UK) (2006) *Statement on the Use of Automated External Defibrillators (Aeds) Until Re-programming to be Compliant with Guidelines 2005.* Resuscitation Council (UK), 2006.

Resuscitation Council (UK) (2009) *Guidance for Safer Handling During Resuscitation in Healthcare Settings.* Resuscitation Council (UK), London.

Resuscitation Council (UK) (2011) *Advanced Life Support,* 6th edn. Resuscitation Council (UK), London.

Resuscitation Council (UK) (2012) *Medical Emergencies and Resuscitation Standards for Clinical Practice and Training for Dental Practitioners and Dental Care Professionals in General Dental Practice.* Resuscitation Council (UK), London.

Tunstall-Pedoe H, Bailey L, Chamberlain D *et al.* (1992) Survey of 3765 cardiopulmonary resuscitations in British hospitals (the BRESUS study): methods and overall results. *BMJ*; 304:1347–1351.

Yokoyama T, Yoshida K, Suwa K (2008) Efficacy of external cardiac compression in a dental chair. *Resuscitation*; 79(1):175–176.

Chapter 10

Airway management and ventilation

INTRODUCTION

Failure of the circulation for 3–4 minutes (less if the patient is initially hypox-aemic) can lead to irreversible cerebral damage. Restarting the heart following a cardiac arrest may not be possible without adequate reoxygenation (Resuscitation Council (UK), 2011).

Patients who require resuscitation often have airway obstruction, usually secondary to loss of consciousness, but sometimes airway obstruction may be the primary cause of cardiorespiratory arrest (Deakin *et al.*, 2010). Airway obstruction can be subtle and is often undetected by healthcare professionals (Deakin *et al.*, 2010).

Dental practitioners must be competent at basic airway management and ventilation. Whatever the cause, prompt recognition and effective treatment of airway obstruction is essential, particularly during resuscitation as an open and clear airway is essential to help ensure adequate ventilation.

The aim of this chapter is to understand the principles of airway management and ventilation.

LEARNING OUTCOMES

At the end of the chapter, the reader will be able to:

- List the causes of airway obstruction
- Outline the recognition of airway obstruction
- Describe simple techniques to open and clear the airway
- Discuss the use of an oropharyngeal airway
- Discuss the principles of ventilation
- Outline the treatment of foreign body airway obstruction

Basic Guide to Medical Emergencies in the Dental Practice, Second Edition. Phil Jevon.
© 2014 John Wiley & Sons, Ltd. Published 2014 by John Wiley & Sons, Ltd.
Companion website: www.wiley.com\go\jevon\medicalemergencies

CAUSES OF AIRWAY OBSTRUCTION

Causes of airway obstruction include:

- *Displaced tongue* – causes include unconsciousness, sedation, cardiac arrest and trauma;
- *Fluid* – e.g. vomit, secretions and blood;
- *Foreign body* – e.g. dentures;
- *Laryngeal oedema* – causes include anaphylaxis and infection;
- *Bronchospasm* – causes include asthma, foreign body and anaphylaxis;
- *Pulmonary oedema* – causes include cardiac failure, anaphylaxis and near drowning (Jevon, 2006a).

RECOGNITION OF AIRWAY OBSTRUCTION

Whatever the cause of airway obstruction, prompt recognition and effective management are essential. Recognition is best achieved by following the familiar 'look, listen and feel' approach (Resuscitation Council (UK), 2011).

- *Look* for movements of the chest and abdomen;
- *Listen* at the mouth and nose for airflow;
- *Feel* at the mouth and nose for airflow.

Airway obstruction can be partial or complete, and can occur at any level from the nose and mouth down to the trachea (Jevon, 2006a).

Partial airway obstruction

Partial airway obstruction is usually characterised by noisy breathing.

- *Gurgling* – presence of fluid, e.g. secretions in the main airways;
- *Snoring* – partial occlusion of the pharynx by the tongue;
- *Inspiratory stridor* – upper airway obstruction (at or above the level of the larynx), e.g. foreign body, laryngeal oedema;
- *Expiratory wheeze* – lower airway obstruction, e.g. asthma.

Complete airway obstruction

Complete airway obstruction in a patient who is making respiratory efforts is characterised by paradoxical chest and abdominal movements ('see-saw' breathing) – on trying to breathe in, the chest is drawn inwards and the abdomen expands, the opposite happening when trying to breathe out (Resuscitation Council (UK), 2011). Use of accessory muscles, e.g. neck and shoulder muscles, may also be evident.

AIRWAY MANAGEMENT AND VENTILATION

SIMPLE TECHNIQUES TO OPEN AND CLEAR THE AIRWAY

Head tilt, chin lift and jaw thrust are three manoeuvres that can improve the patency of the airway, which has been obstructed by the tongue or other upper airway structures, e.g. soft palate and epiglottis (Deakin *et al.*, 2010). As regurgitation of gastric contents and vomiting commonly occurs during resuscitation, suction is regularly required and proficiency in applying it is essential (Jevon, 2006a).

Head tilt, chin lift

The head tilt, chin lift manoeuvre (Figure 10.1) is considered, the most effective method of opening the airway of an unconscious patient (Jevon, 2009). In basic life support it can achieve airway patency in 91% of cases (Guildner *et al.*, 1976). By stretching the anterior tissues of the neck, it displaces the tongue forwards away from the posterior pharyngeal wall and lifts the epiglottis from the laryngeal opening (Jevon, 2009). A cushion under the head and shoulders can help to maintain this position.

To perform head tilt and chin lift:

- Place one hand on the patient's forehead and gently tilt the head back;
- Place the fingertips of the other hand under the point of the patient's chin and lift the chin upwards.

Source: Jevon (2006a)

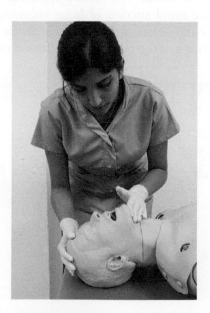

Figure 10.1 Head tilt, chin lift manoeuvre.

AIRWAY MANAGEMENT AND
VENTILATION

Jaw thrust

The jaw thrust manoeuvre (Figure 10.2) is an alternative method to open the airway. It is recommended in patients with a suspected cervical spine injury (Jevon, 2009), as head tilt may aggravate the injury and damage the spinal cord (Donaldson *et al.*, 1997). When used in these patients, it should be accompanied by manual in-line immobilisation of the head and neck by an assistant (Lennarson *et al.*, 2001). However, if life-threatening airway obstruction persists, despite the application of effective jaw thrust or chin lift, head tilt should be performed gradually more and more until airway patency is achieved. The establishment of a clear airway takes priority over concerns about potential injury to the cervical spine (Deakin *et al.*, 2010).

To perform a jaw thrust:

- Using the index fingers, positioned just proximal to the angles of the jaw, displace the mandible anteriorly (together with the tongue);
- Using the thumbs, apply pressure on the chin to help open the mouth.

Source: Jevon (2006a)

Suction

When obstruction is caused by vomit, secretions, etc., simple basic life support manoeuvres such as placing the patient in the lateral position and finger sweeps may help to clear the airway. The suction apparatus by the dental chair (Figure 10.3) can provide rapid suction of large volumes of fluid from the mouth and pharynx. A hand-held portable suction device (see Chapter 1) is useful for some situations, e.g. if the patient has collapsed in the waiting room.

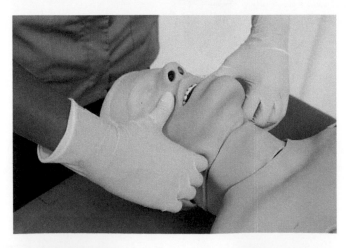

Figure 10.2 Jaw thrust manoeuvre.

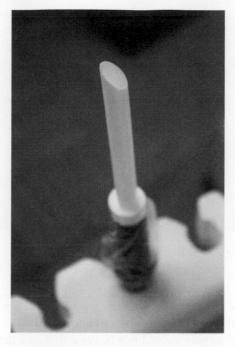

Figure 10.3 Suction apparatus.

Dentures

Well-fitting dentures should be left in place because they will help to maintain the normal shape of the face, facilitating an adequate seal when ventilating using a bag, valve or mask device. However, displaced or broken dentures should be removed (Jevon, 2006a).

USE OF OROPHARYNGEAL AIRWAY

The oropharyngeal airway is a useful adjunct because it can provide an artificial passage to airflow by separating the posterior pharyngeal wall from the tongue.

Oropharyngeal airway

The oropharyngeal airway (Figure 10.4) can be used when there is obstruction of the upper airway due to the displacement of the tongue backwards and when glossopharyngeal and laryngeal reflexes are absent, e.g. during cardiopulmonary resuscitation.

AIRWAY MANAGEMENT AND VENTILATION

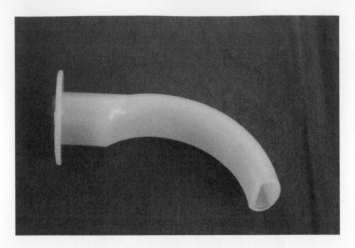

Figure 10.4 Oropharyngeal airway.

Cautions
- An oropharyngeal airway should not be used in a patient who is not unconscious as it may induce vomiting and laryngospasm.
- An oropharyngeal airway should not be regarded as a definitive airway.
- The appropriate size of airway should always be estimated.
- The correct insertion technique should be adopted to minimise complications.

Estimating the correct size
It is important to estimate the correct size. An oropharyngeal airway that is too big may occlude the airway by displacing the epiglottis (Jevon, 2009), may hinder the use of a face mask and may damage laryngeal structures, while one that is too small may occlude the airway by pushing the tongue back.

An appropriately sized airway is one that holds the tongue in the normal anatomical position and follows its natural curvature (Jevon, 2006b). The curved body of the oropharyngeal airway is designed to fit over the back of the tongue.

The correct size is one that equates to the vertical distance from the angle of the jaw to the incisors (Resuscitation Council (UK), 2011); this can be estimated by placing the airway against the face and measuring it from the patient's incisors to the angle of the jaw. A variety of different sizes are available, though normally sizes 2, 3 and 4 are adequate for small, medium and large adults, respectively (Resuscitation Council (UK), 2011).

Procedure for insertion

The correct insertion technique should be used in order to avoid unnecessary trauma to the delicate tissues in the mouth and so as not to inadvertently block the airway.

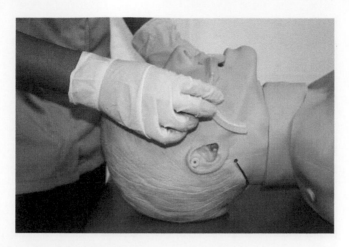

Figure 10.5 Insertion of oropharyngeal airway: estimating the correct size.

- Ensure the patient is in a supine position.
- Don gloves (if available).
- Clear the patient's airway, suction the mouth if necessary.
- Estimate the correct size by placing the airway against the patient's face and measuring it from the angle of the jaw to the incisors (Figure 10.5).
- If possible, lubricate the airway before insertion (practically, in the emergency situation, this is rarely done).
- Open the patient's mouth, clear the airway by suction if necessary and insert the airway in the inverted position (Figure 10.6) (the curved part of the airway will help depress the tongue and prevent it from being pushed posteriorly).

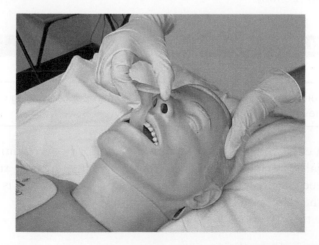

Figure 10.6 Insertion of oropharyngeal airway: insert the airway in the inverted position initially.

AIRWAY MANAGEMENT AND VENTILATION

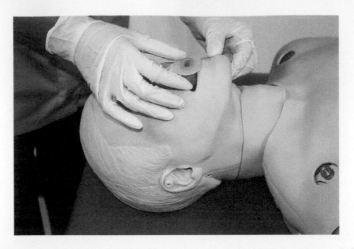

Figure 10.7 Insertion of oropharyngeal airway: as it passes over the soft palate, rotate the airway through 180 degrees.

- As it passes over the soft palate, rotate the airway through 180 degrees (Figure 10.7).
- After insertion, confirm that the airway has been positioned correctly: the patient's airway should be improved and the flattened, reinforced section should be positioned between the patient's teeth, or between the gums, if edentulous (Resuscitation Council (UK), 2011).
- Closely monitor the patency and position of the airway; it can become blocked by the tongue or epiglottis and can become wedged into the vallecula (Marsh *et al.*, 1991). Vomit, secretions and blood can also compromise its patency.

Source: Jevon (2006b)

PRINCIPLES OF VENTILATION

> The most common cause of failure to ventilate is improper positioning of the head and chin (Jevon, 2006c)

Although chest compressions are now given priority over ventilations during the initial resuscitation sequence, effective ventilations are still required and are indeed essential in prolonged arrests if cerebral function is to be maintained and the chance of survival is to be optimised.

There are three methods for ventilation:

- Mouth-to-mouth ventilation;
- Mouth-to-mask ventilation;
- Ventilation using a self-inflating bag (bag/valve/mask device).

AIRWAY MANAGEMENT AND VENTILATION

Mouth-to-mouth ventilation

It should not be necessary to perform mouth-to-mouth resuscitation in the dental practice. At the very least, a pocket mask should always be immediately available. However, for completeness, the procedure will now be described.

Mouth-to-mouth ventilation is a quick, effective way to provide adequate oxygenation and ventilation in a patient who is not breathing. However, it is only possible to deliver 16–17% oxygen to the patient; a ventilatory device with supplementary oxygen should be used as soon as practically possible.

Barrier devices

Both healthcare workers and laypersons are often reluctant to perform mouth-to-mouth ventilation, most commonly due to a fear of contracting HIV (Brenner *et al.*, 1997; Resuscitation Council (UK), 2011). Consequently, a variety of barrier devices is available (Figure 10.8); face masks with one-way valves prevent the transmission of bacteria, while face shields are less effective.

Procedure for mouth-to-mouth ventilation

1. Ensure the patient is supine. In a cardiac arrest, 30 chest compressions should have been performed first before delivering 2 ventilations (ratio 30:2).
2. Kneel in a comfortable position with the knees, a shoulder width apart, at the side of the patient at the level of his nose and mouth (a wider base will be required to undertake compressions if only one person is performing CPR) (Resuscitation Council (UK), 2009).
3. Rest back to sit on the heels in the low-kneeling position (Resuscitation Council (UK), 2009).
4. Apply a barrier device, if one is available and, if trained to do so.
5. Bend forwards from the hips, leaning down towards the patient's nose and mouth (Resuscitation Council (UK), 2009).

AIRWAY MANAGEMENT AND VENTILATION

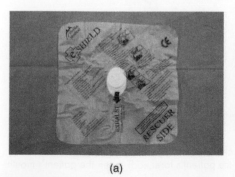

(a)

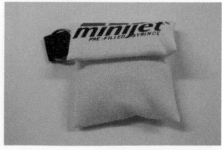

(b)

Figure 10.8 (a, b) Barrier devices.

6. While maintaining head tilt and chin lift, pinch the soft part of the patient's nose (use the index finger and thumb of the hand on the patient's forehead), open the patient's mouth and take a normal breath in (Figure 10.9).
7. Place your lips around the patient's mouth, ensuring a good seal, and blow into the patient's mouth over 1 second and watch for chest to rise.
8. While still maintaining head tilt and chin lift, remove your mouth and watch for chest to fall. Repeat the procedure and then ensure 30 chest compressions are performed.
9. If the initial ventilation does not achieve chest rise as in normal breathing, before the next attempt, check the patient's mouth and remove any obstruction and recheck to ensure adequate head tilt and chin lift and ensure adequate seal. Only attempt 2 ventilations before 30 chest compressions are performed again.
10. If the patient is in the dental chair (its height should already have been adjusted so that the patient is level between the knee and mid-thigh of the dental practitioner performing chest compressions): stand at the side facing the patient, level with his nose and mouth and bend forwards from the hips to minimise flexion of the spine (Resuscitation Council (UK), 2009).

Source: Resuscitation Council (UK), 2009, Resuscitation Council (UK), 2011, Jevon, 2006b

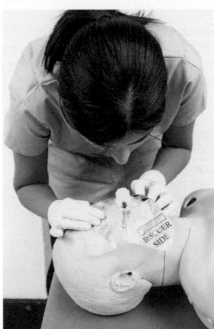

Figure 10.9 While maintaining head tilt and chin lift, pinch the soft part of the patient's nose (use the index finger and thumb of the hand on the patient's forehead), open the patient's mouth and take a normal breath in.

Ineffective delivery of rescue breaths

If it is difficult to deliver effective breaths:

- Ensure adequate head tilt and chin lift;
- Check the patient's mouth and remove any obstruction;
- Ensure a good seal between your mouth and the patient's mouth;
- Ensure the patient's nose is pinched during ventilation.

Minimising gastric inflation

Gastric inflation is commonly associated with mouth-to-mouth ventilation, occurring when the pressure in the oesophagus exceeds the opening pressure of the lower oesophageal sphincter, resulting in the sphincter opening (Jevon, 2009). During CPR, the oesophageal sphincter relaxes, thus increasing the likelihood of gastric inflation (Jevon, 2009).

Excessive tidal volumes or inspiratory flows can generate excessive airway pressures that can lead to gastric inflation and the subsequent risk of regurgitation and aspiration of gastric contents (Deakin *et al.*, 2010). It is therefore recommended to deliver each ventilation over 1 second, with sufficient volume to achieve chest rise, but avoiding rapid and forceful ventilations (Resuscitation Council (UK), 2011).

Mouth-to-mask ventilation (pocket mask)

The pocket mask (Figure 10.10) is an excellent, first response device. It is transparent, thus enabling prompt detection of vomit or blood in the patient's airway. A one-way valve directs the patient's expired air away from the nurse.

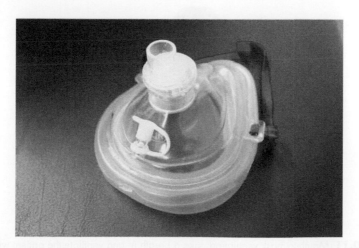

Figure 10.10 Pocket mask.

Most pocket masks have an oxygen connector for the attachment of supplementary oxygen (15 l/min), enabling an inspired oxygen concentration of approximately 50% to be achieved. If there is no oxygen connector, supplementary oxygen can still be added by placing the oxygen tubing underneath one side of the mask and pressing down to achieve a seal (Deakin *et al.*, 2010).

Procedure for mouth-to-mask ventilation – patient on the floor

1. Don gloves (if available).
2. Kneel behind the patient's head, ensuring the knees are a shoulder-width apart (if working alone, kneel at the side of the patient level with his nose and mouth) (Resuscitation Council (UK), 2009).
3. Rest back to sit on the knees and adopt a low-kneeling position (Resuscitation Council (UK), 2009).
4. Bend forwards from the hips, leaning down towards the patient's face and resting the elbows on your legs to support your weight (Resuscitation Council (UK), 2009).
5. If available, attach oxygen to the oxygen connector on the mask at a rate of 15 l/min. If there is no oxygen connector, place the oxygen tubing underneath one side of the mask and press down to achieve a seal (Deakin *et al.*, 2010).
6. Apply the mask to the patient's face; press down with the thumbs and lift the chin into the mask by applying pressure behind the angles of the jaw.
7. Take a breath in and ventilate the patient with sufficient air to cause visible chest rise (Figure 10.11). Each ventilation should last 1 second.

Source: Resuscitation Council (UK) (2009), Resuscitation Council (UK) (2011), Jevon (2006b)

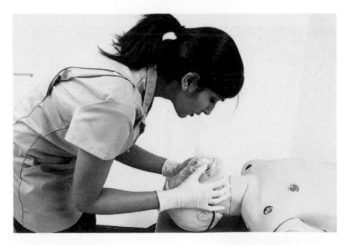

Figure 10.11 Mouth-to-mask ventilation: take a breath in and ventilate the patient with sufficient air to cause visible chest rise.

AIRWAY MANAGEMENT AND VENTILATION

Procedure for mouth-to-mask ventilation – patient in the dental chair

- Don gloves (if available).
- Ensure the patient is supine in the chair (its height should already have been adjusted so that the patient is level between the knee and mid-thigh of the person performing chest compressions).
- While your colleague performs chest compressions, sit on the dentist's stool behind the head end of the chair, facing the patient.
- If available, attach oxygen to the oxygen connector on the mask at a rate of 15 l/min. If there is no oxygen connector, place the oxygen tubing underneath one side of the mask and pressing down to achieve a seal (Deakin *et al.*, 2010).
- Apply the mask to the patient's face; press down with the thumbs and lift the chin into the mask by applying pressure behind the angles of the jaw.
- Bend forwards from the hips, leaning down towards the patient's face and resting the elbows on your legs to support your weight (Resuscitation Council (UK), 2009).
- Take a breath in and ventilate the patient with sufficient air to cause visible chest rise. Each ventilation should last 1 second.
- Always adopt a comfortable position for ventilation and avoid static postures (Resuscitation Council (UK), 2009); ideally sit on the dentist's stool.

Source: Resuscitation Council (UK) (2009), Resuscitation Council (UK) (2011), Jevon (2006b)

If working alone when performing mouth- to- mask ventilation, stand at the side facing the patient, level with his nose and mouth, and bend forwards from the hips to minimise flexion of the spine (Resuscitation Council (UK), 2009)

Bag-mask ventilation

The bag-mask (self-inflating bag) (Figure 10.12) device allows the delivery of higher concentrations of oxygen. If an oxygen reservoir bag is attached, with an oxygen flow rate of 10 l/min, an inspired oxygen concentration of approximately 85% can be achieved (Resuscitation Council (UK), 2011).

However, its use by a single person requires considerable skill. When used with a face mask, it can be difficult to achieve a seal with the mask, maintain an open airway and squeeze the bag (Jevon, 2009). A two-person technique is therefore recommended, one person to open the airway and ensure a good seal with the mask, while the other squeezes the bag (Resuscitation Council (UK), 2011).

AIRWAY MANAGEMENT AND VENTILATION

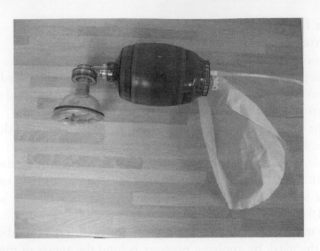

Figure 10.12 Self-inflating bag.

Procedure for bag-mask ventilation – patient on the floor

1. Don gloves (if available).
2. Select an appropriately sized mask, i.e. one that comfortably covers the mouth and nose but does not cover the eyes or override the chin.
3. Ensure the oxygen reservoir bag is attached to the self-inflating bag and connect oxygen at a flow rate of 15 l/min (Resuscitation Council (UK), 2011).
4. Kneel behind the patient's head, ensuring the knees are a shoulder-width apart (Resuscitation Council (UK), 2009).
5. Rest back to sit on the heels and adopt a low-kneeling position (Resuscitation Council (UK), 2009).
6. Rest your elbows on your legs to support your weight; adopt a comfortable position, e.g. bend forwards or remain upright (Resuscitation Council (UK), 2009).
7. Tilt the patient's head back; apply the mask to the face, pressing down on it with the thumbs. Lift the chin into the mask by applying pressure behind the angles of the jaw. An open airway and an adequate face-to-mask seal should now be achieved. A cushion under the head and shoulders can help to maintain this position.
8. Ask a colleague to kneel to the side, adopting the same stance as described above.
9. After the delivery of 30 chest compressions, ask your colleague to deliver two ventilations, squeezing the self-inflating bag (not the oxygen reservoir bag) sufficiently to cause visible chest rise (Figure 10.13). Each ventilation should be delivered over 1 second.
10. Observe for chest rise and fall. If the chest does not rise, re-check the patency of the airway; slight readjustment may be all that is required.

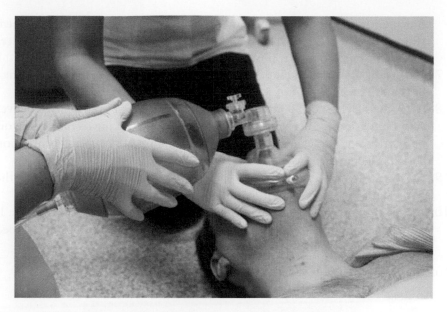

Figure 10.13 Patient on the floor: ventilation with a self-inflating bag.

11. Adopt a comfortable position for ventilation and avoid static postures. It may be helpful to support your weight by resting your elbows on the bed (Resuscitation Council (UK), 2009).

Source: Resuscitation Council (UK) (2009), (2011), Jevon (2006b)

Procedure for bag-mask ventilation – patient in the dental chair

1. Don gloves (if available).
2. Ensure the patient is supine. The height of the chair should already have been adjusted so that the patient is level between the knee and mid-thigh of the person performing chest compressions (Resuscitation Council (UK), 2009).
3. Adopt a comfortable position for ventilation. Sit on the dentist's stool behind the head end of the chair, facing the patient. It may be helpful to support your weight by resting your elbows on your knees (Resuscitation Council (UK), 2009).
4. Select an appropriately sized mask, i.e. one that comfortably covers the mouth and nose but does not cover the eyes or override the chin.
5. Ensure the oxygen reservoir bag is attached to the self-inflating bag and connect oxygen at a flow rate of 15 l/min (Resuscitation Council (UK), 2011).
6. Tilt the patient's head back; apply the mask to the face, pressing down on it with the thumbs. Lift the chin into the mask by applying pressure behind

AIRWAY MANAGEMENT AND VENTILATION

the angles of the jaw. An open airway and an adequate face-to-mask seal should now be achieved. A small cushion under the head and shoulders can help to maintain this position.

7. Ask a colleague to stand at the side facing the patient's head, with the feet in the walk/stand position (Resuscitation Council (UK), 2009).
8. After the delivery of 30 chest compressions, ask your colleague to deliver two ventilations, squeezing the self-inflating bag (not the oxygen reservoir bag) sufficiently to cause visible chest rise (Figure 10.14). Each ventilation should be delivered over 1 second.
9. Observe for chest rise and fall. If the chest does not rise, re-check the patency of the airway; slight readjustment may be all that is required.
10. Adopt a comfortable position for ventilation and avoid static postures. It may be helpful to support your weight by resting your elbows on the bed (Resuscitation Council (UK), 2009).

Source: Resuscitation Council (UK) (2009), (2011), Jevon (2006b)

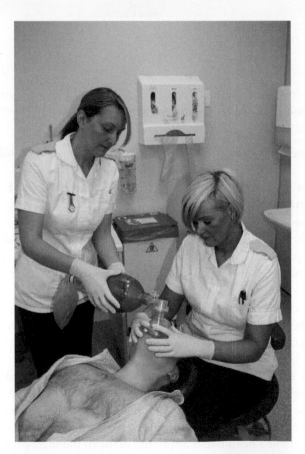

Figure 10.14 Patient in the dental chair: ventilation with a self-inflating bag.

Minimising gastric inflation

Excessive tidal volumes or inspiratory flows can generate excessive airway pressures that can lead to gastric inflation and the subsequent risk of regurgitation and aspiration of gastric contents (Resuscitation Council (UK), 2011). It is therefore recommended to deliver each ventilation over 1 second, with sufficient volume to achieve chest rise, but avoiding rapid and forceful ventilations (Koster *et al.*, 2010).

Ineffective ventilations

If ventilations fail to achieve chest rise:

- ensure adequate head tilt and chin lift;
- recheck the patient's mouth and remove any obstruction;
- ensure there is a good seal between the mask and the patient's face.

TREATMENT OF FOREIGN BODY AIRWAY OBSTRUCTION

Foreign body airway obstruction (choking) is a life-threatening emergency. As most such events are associated with eating, they are commonly witnessed, thus providing an opportunity for early intervention while the patient is still conscious (Resuscitation Council (UK), 2011). Case reports have demonstrated the effectiveness of back blows, abdominal thrusts and chest thrusts for the treatment of foreign body airway obstruction (ILCOR, 2005), successful treatment often requiring more than one particular intervention (Redding, 1979).

Incidence

Foreign body airway obstruction is an uncommon, yet potentially treatable, cause of accidental death (Fingerhut *et al.*, 1998). Each year in the United Kingdom approximately 16,000 adults and children receive treatment in the emergency department for foreign body airway obstruction (Resuscitation Council (UK), 2011); less than 1% of these are fatal (Department of Trade and Industry, 1999a). In adults, the commonest cause of foreign body airway obstruction is food, e.g. meat, poultry and fish (Department of Trade and Industry, 1999a); in children half of the cases are caused by food (usually sweets) and half by such items as small toys and coins (Department of Trade and Industry, 1999b).

Recognition of foreign body airway obstruction

Complete foreign body airway obstruction is often characterised by a sudden inability to talk, maximal respiratory effort, development of cyanosis and

AIRWAY MANAGEMENT AND VENTILATION

clutching of the neck. In partial airway obstruction, the patient will be distressed, may cough and may have a wheeze. In complete airway obstruction, the casualty will be unable to speak, breathe or cough and will eventually collapse and become unconscious. Always ask the patient 'are you choking?' (Koster *et al.*, 2010). If he responds 'yes' by nodding his head without speaking, this indicates severe airway obstruction requiring urgent treatment (American Heart Association, 2005).

If the patient is choking, but able to breathe, encourage him to cough. If the patient is choking and is unable to breathe or is displaying signs of becoming weak or stops breathing or coughing, immediate intervention is required.

Procedure for treatment of foreign body airway obstruction

- Stand at side, slightly behind the patient.
- Support his chest with one hand and lean him well forwards. This will help ensure that if the foreign body is dislodged, it will drop out of the mouth instead of slipping further down the airway.
- Deliver up to five back blows between the scapulae using the heel of the hand (Figure 10.15). After each back blow, check to see if it has been successful at relieving the obstruction.

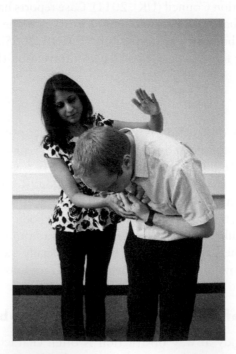

Figure 10.15 Choking: back slaps.

- If the back blows fail, proceed to abdominal thrusts.
- Stand behind the patient, placing both arms around his upper abdomen.
- Lean the patient forwards.
- Place a clenched fist between the patient's umbilicus and xiphisternum and clasp it with the other hand (Figure 10.16).
- Deliver up to five sharp thrusts to the abdomen, inwards and upwards.
- If the obstruction remains, continue alternating five back blows with five chest abdominal thrusts.

   If the patient loses consciousness:

- carefully support him to the ground;
- immediately call 999 for an ambulance;
- start CPR, 30 chest compressions first (even if there is a pulse) – chest compressions may relieve the obstruction (Koster *et al.*, 2010).

Chest thrusts versus abdominal thrusts

Chest thrusts can generate higher airway pressures than abdominal thrusts (Guilder *et al.*, 1976; Ruben and Macnaughton, 1978). If a patient with a foreign body airway obstruction loses consciousness, CPR should be started, as chest thrusts are almost identical to chest compressions (Resuscitation Council

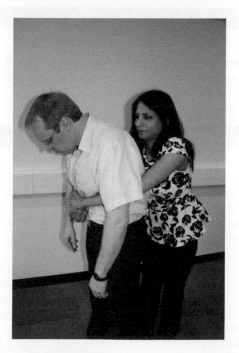

Figure 10.16 Choking: abdominal thrusts.

AIRWAY MANAGEMENT AND VENTILATION

(UK), 2011). Then each time the airway is opened to provide ventilations, check the mouth in case the foreign body has been dislodged.

Finger sweeps

The routine use of a finger sweep to clear the airway in the absence of visible airway obstruction has yet to be evaluated (Hartrey and Bingham, 1995; Elam *et al.*, 1960). Finger sweeps have been reported to cause harm to both the patient (Resuscitation Council (UK), 2011) and the rescuer (ILCOR, 2005). Blind finger sweeps are not recommended; only manually remove a foreign body in the airway if it can be seen (Koster *et al.*, 2010).

Follow-up

Following successful treatment, a foreign body may still be present in the airways: therefore if the patient has dysphagia, has a persistent cough or complains of having something 'stuck in his throat', he should be referred to a doctor (Koster *et al.*, 2010).

As abdominal thrusts can cause serious internal injury, e.g. rupture or laceration of abdominal or thoracic viscera, patients who have been treated with abdominal thrusts must be referred to a doctor (ILCOR, 2005).

CONCLUSION

Effective airway management and ventilation are essential if oxygen supply to the brain is to be maintained during cardiopulmonary resuscitation. This chapter has described the principles of basic airway management and ventilation.

REFERENCES

American Heart Association (2005) 2005 American Heart Association Guidelines for cardiopulmonary resuscitation and emergency cardiovascular care. *Circulation*; 112(24 suppl):IV1–203.

Brenner B, Van D, Cheng D, Lazar E (1997) Determinants of reluctance to perform CPR among residents and applicants: the impact of experience on helping behaviour. *Resuscitation*; 35:203–211.

Deakin C, Nolan J, Soar J *et al.* (2010) European Resuscitation Council Guidelines for Resuscitation 2010: section 4. adult advanced life support. *Resuscitation*; 81(10):1305–1352.

Department of Trade and Industry (1999a) Choking. *Home and Leisure Accident Report*. Department of Trade and Industry, London.

Department of Trade and Industry (1999b) *Choking Risks for Children*. Department of Trade and Industry, London.

Donaldson W, Heil B, Donaldson V, Silvaggio V (1997) The effect of airway manoeuvres on the unstable C1-C2 segment: a cadaver study. *Spine*; 22:1215–1218.

Elam J, Ruben A, Greene D (1960) Resuscitation of drowning victims. *Journal of American Medical Association*; 174:13–16.

Fingerhut L, Cox C, Warner M (1998) International comparative analysis of injury mortality: findings from the ICE on injury statistics. International collaborative effort on injury statistics. *Advance Data*; 12:1–20.

Guildner C, Williams D, Subitch T (1976) Airway obstructed by foreign material: the Heimlich maneuver. Journal of the American College of Emergency Physicians; 5:675–677.

Hartrey R, Bingham R (1995) Pharyngeal trauma as a result of blind finger sweeps in the choking child. *Journal of Accident and Emergency Medicine*; 12:52–54.

ILCOR (2005) Part 2 adult basic life support 2005 international consensus on cardiopulmonary resuscitation and emergency cardiovascular care science with treatment recommendations. *Resuscitation*; 67:187–200.

Jevon P (2006a) Resuscitation skills – part 2: clearing the airway. *Nursing Times*; 102(26):26–27.

Jevon P (2006b) Resuscitation skills – part 3: basic airway management. *Nursing Times*; 102(27):26–27.

Jevon P (2006c) Mask ventilation. *Nursing Times*; 102(38):28–29.

Jevon P (2009) *Advanced Cardiac Life Support*, 2nd edn. Wiley-Blackwell, Oxford.

Koster R, Baubin M, Bossaert L *et al.* (2010) European resuscitation council guidelines for resuscitation 2010 section 2. Adult basic life support and use of automated external defibrillators. *Resuscitation*; 81(10):1277–1292.

Lennarson P, Smith D, Sawin P *et al.* (2001) Cervical spine motion during intubation: efficacy of stabilization maneuvers in the setting of complete segmental instability. *Journal of Neurosurgery*; 94:265–270.

Marsh A, Nunn J, Taylor S, Charlesworth C (1991) Airway obstruction associated with the use of the Guedel airway. *British Journal of Anaesthesia*; 67:517–523.

Redding J (1979) The choking controversy: critique of evidence of the Heimlich maneuver. *Critical Care Medicine*; 7:475–479.

Resuscitation Council (UK) (2009) *Guidance for Safer Handling During Resuscitation in Healthcare Settings*. Resuscitation Council (UK), London.

Resuscitation Council (UK) (2011) *Advanced Life Support*, 6th edn. Resuscitation Council (UK), London.

Ruben H, Macnaughton F (1978) The treatment of food-choking. *Practitioner*; 221:725–729.

AIRWAY MANAGEMENT AND VENTILATION

Chapter 11
Automated external defibrillation

INTRODUCTION

Defibrillation is the delivery of an electrical current across the myocardium of significant magnitude to depolarise a critical mass of the myocardium simultaneously to enable the restoration of organised electrical activity. A key component in the chain of survival (see Chapter 1 and Figure 1.1), defibrillation is one of only two interventions that have been shown unequivocally to improve long-term survival following a cardiac arrest, the other being basic life support (Resuscitation Council (UK), 2011).

The modern automated external defibrillator (AED) abolishes the need for the operator to have ECG interpretation skills. Spoken and/or visual prompts guide the operator through the safe use of the AED. As minimal training is required, it can be used by a wide range of personnel, including dental practice staff. The Resuscitation Council (UK) (2012) now recommends that every dental practice should have immediate access to a defibrillator. If required, defibrillation should be undertaken by dental staff before the arrival of the paramedics.

The aim of this chapter is to understand the principles of automated external defibrillation.

LEARNING OUTCOMES

At the end of this chapter, the reader will be able to:

- Recognise ventricular fibrillation
- Discuss the physiology of defibrillation
- Outline the factors affecting successful defibrillation
- Discuss the safety issues related to defibrillation
- Describe the procedure for automated external defibrillation

---

Basic Guide to Medical Emergencies in the Dental Practice, Second Edition. Phil Jevon.
© 2014 John Wiley & Sons, Ltd. Published 2014 by John Wiley & Sons, Ltd.
Companion website: www.wiley.com\go\jevon\medicalemergencies

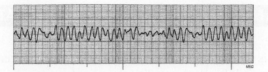

Figure 11.1 Ventricular fibrillation.

VENTRICULAR FIBRILLATION

'The cardiac pump is thrown out of gear, and the last of its vital energy is dissipated in a violent and prolonged turmoil of fruitless activity in the ventricular walls' (McWilliam, 1889).

In ventricular fibrillation (Figure 11.1), the myocardium is depolarising at random, resulting in uncoordinated electrical activity, with subsequent loss of cardiac output and cardiac arrest. Causes include myocardial ischaemia, electrolyte imbalance, hypothermia, drug toxicity and electric shock.

Ventricular fibrillation is the commonest primary arrhythmia at the onset of cardiac arrest in adults (Resuscitation Council (UK), 2011). It is an eminently treatable arrhythmia, with most eventual survivors of a cardiac arrest belonging to this group (Tunstall-Pedoe *et al.*, 1992).

Early defibrillation is the definitive treatment; the chances of success decline substantially (7–10%) with each passing minute of delay to defibrillation (Waalewijn *et al.*, 2001). There is a slower decline if there is adequate basic life support (Resuscitation Council (UK), 2011).

PHYSIOLOGY OF DEFIBRILLATION

The heart can respond to an extrinsic electrical impulse just as it can respond to an impulse from the sino-atrial node or from an ectopic focus. It is thought that successful defibrillation occurs when a critical mass of myocardium is depolarised by the passage of an electric current (Resuscitation Council (UK), 2011); if 75–90% of myocardial cells are in the repolarisation phase when the current is removed, successful defibrillation occurs and the sino-atrial node or another intrinsic pacemaker can then regain control.

Success will depend on the actual current flow rather than shock energy. This current flow is influenced by transthoracic impedance (resistance of the chest tissues), electrode position and shock energy delivered. Only a small proportion of the energy delivered actually reaches the myocardium; an effective defibrillation technique is essential to optimise the chances of successful defibrillation.

FACTORS AFFECTING SUCCESSFUL DEFIBRILLATION

If defibrillation is to be successful, sufficient electrical current needs to pass through the chest and depolarise a critical mass of myocardium. Transthoracic impedance and incorrect positioning of the adhesive pad electrodes are two key factors that can affect successful defibrillation.

Transthoracic impedance

Transthoracic impedance is the resistance to the flow of current through the chest; the greater the resistance, the lesser the current flow. The contact between the adhesive pad electrodes and the skin can be poor if the patient has a hairy chest, trapping air between the electrode and the skin; this can result in increased transthoracic impedance, reduced defibrillation efficacy and arcing (sparks) causing burns to the patient's chest (Deakin *et al.*, 2010).

If the patient has a hairy chest and a razor is immediately available, quickly remove hair from the area where the adhesive pad electrodes are going to be placed, but if a razor is not immediately available, do not delay defibrillation (Resuscitation Council (UK), 2011).

Incorrect positioning of the adhesive pad electrodes

The adhesive pad electrodes should be placed in the correct positions on the chest wall to maximise the current flow through the myocardium. It is important to follow the manufacturer's instructions – most adhesive pad electrodes will have a diagram to guide correct placement (Figure 11.2). Adhesive pad electrodes are generally placed, one on the anterior chest, just to the right of the sternum (not over the sternum) below the right clavicle, the other in the

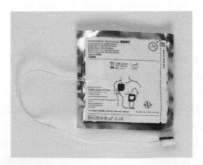

Figure 11.2 Adhesive pad electrodes.

AUTOMATED EXTERNAL DEFIBRILLATION

mid-axillary line near the apex of the heart. In women, breast tissue should be avoided as this can increase transthoracic impedance.

The accuracy of electrode placement by healthcare staff has been questioned, and care should be taken to ensure their correct placement following the manufacturer's instructions.

SAFETY ISSUES AND DEFIBRILLATION

General safety issues

- Confirm cardiac arrest.
- Avoid direct and indirect contact with the patient. All personnel should be well away from the dental chair; no one should be touching the patient or anything attached to the dental chair.
- Ensure that no personnel are standing in water which is in contact with the chair.
- Temporarily remove oxygen delivery device at least 1 metre away from the patient's chest (Resuscitation Council (UK), 2011).
- Shout 'stand clear' and check all personnel are safely clear, prior to defibrillation. No person should be touching the patient or anything in contact with the patient, e.g. bed or drip stand.
- Place the adhesive pad electrodes 12–15 cm away from an implanted pacing unit or implantable cardioverter defibrillator (ICD) (Resuscitation Council (UK), 2011 (most units are sited below the left clavicle, therefore the standard electrode position can be adopted, if below the right clavicle the anterior–posterior paddle position may be necessary).

Safety issues when using adhesive electrode pads

- Ensure that electrode pads are in date.
- Ensure that the patient's chest is wiped dry.
- Shave the chest if necessary (see General safety issues).

PROCEDURE FOR AUTOMATED EXTERNAL DEFIBRILLATION

The following procedure for automated external defibrillation is based on Resuscitation Council (UK) (2011) recommendations and the Resuscitation Council (UK) algorithm for automated external defibrillation (see Figure 9.1).

AUTOMATED EXTERNAL
DEFIBRILLATION

1. Confirm cardiac arrest and ensure a colleague calls 999 for ambulance; if numbers allow, ask someone to wait outside the dental practice to 'flag down' the ambulance.
2. Commence CPR 30 chest compressions:2 ventilations; request the resuscitation equipment and AED.
3. Switch on AED and follow spoken and/or visual prompts.
4. Expose the patient's chest; remove GTN patches (Wrenn, 1990).
5. Prepare the patient's skin as necessary; ensure that the skin is dry and if necessary quickly remove any excess chest hair (if the patient has a hairy chest, the defibrillation electrodes may stick to the hairs resulting in high transthoracic impedance).
6. Apply adhesive pad electrodes to the patient's bare chest following the manufacturer's recommendations; the standard position for the position of the electrodes is one on the anterior chest, just to the right of the sternum (not over the sternum) below the right clavicle, the other in the mid-axillary line approximately level with the fifth intercostal space (Figure 11.3).
7. Stop CPR and ensure nobody is touching the patient during ECG analysis by the AED. This is to prevent artefactual errors during ECG analysis (Resuscitation Council (UK), 2011; Jevon, 2009). Some AEDs require the operator to press an 'analyse' button, while others automatically begin assessment once the adhesive pad electrodes are attached to the patient's chest.

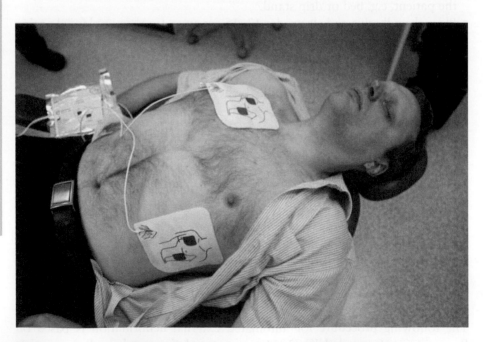

Figure 11.3 Automated external defibrillation: application of adhesive pad electrodes on the chest.

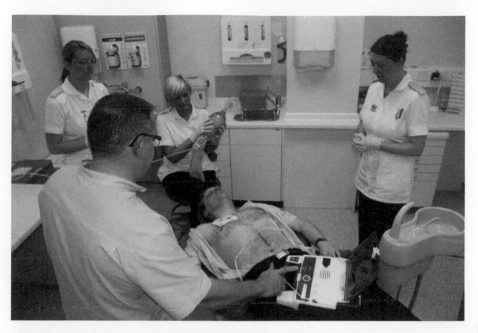

Figure 11.4 Automated external defibrillation: if shock is advised, shout 'stand clear' and perform visual check to ensure that all staff are clear.

8. If shock is advised, shout 'stand clear' and perform visual check to ensure all staff are clear (Figure 11.4).
9. Check all personnel are safely clear before defibrillation. No person should be touching the patient or anything in contact with the patient, e.g. chair or equipment connected to the chair. Request that the ventilatory device and attached oxygen is temporarily removed 1 metre away from the patient (Resuscitation Council (UK), 2011).
10. Press shock button as indicated (if the AED is fully automated, it will deliver the shock automatically) (Figure 11.5).
11. Continue CPR 30 compressions:2 ventilations as guided by the voice/ visual prompts.
12. Following 2 minutes of CPR, the AED will assess again (see step 7 of this section). If a further shock is advised, repeat steps 8–11. If no shock is advised, repeat step 11 if there are no signs of life.

Implantable cardioverter defibrillator

If a patient with an ICD has a cardiac arrest, standard CPR can be carried out without any risks to the team. If the ICD discharges, it will not be detected by those carrying out the CPR. Place the adhesive pad electrodes 12–15 cm away from an implanted pacing unit or ICD (Resuscitation Council (UK), 2011)

AUTOMATED EXTERNAL
DEFIBRILLATION

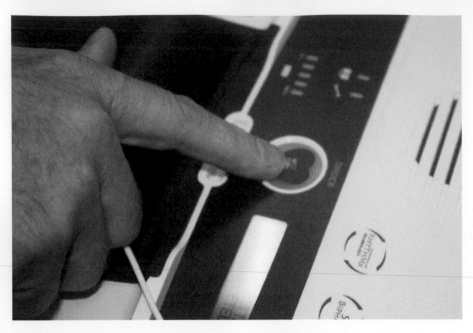

Figure 11.5 Automated external defibrillation: press shock button.

(most units are situated below the left clavicle, therefore the standard electrode position can be adopted; if below the right clavicle, the anterior–posterior paddle position may be necessary).

CONCLUSION

Early defibrillation is a key component in the chain of survival. It has been shown unequivocally to improve long-term survival following a cardiac arrest. It should be delivered promptly, safely and effectively. The Resuscitation Council (UK) (2012) recommends that dental practices should have immediate access to an AED. The principles of automated external defibrillation have been described.

REFERENCES

Deakin C, Nolan J, Sunde K, Koster R (2010) European Resuscitation Council guidelines for resuscitation 2010: Section 3. Electrical therapies: automated external defibrillators, defibrillation, cardioversion and pacing. *Resuscitation*; 81:1293–1804.
McWilliam J (1899) Cardiac failure and sudden death. *BMJ*; I:6–8.

Resuscitation Council (UK) (2011) *Advanced Life Support*, 6th edn. Resuscitation Council (UK), London.

Resuscitation Council (UK) (2012) *Medical Emergencies and Resuscitation Standards for Clinical Practice and Training for Dental Practitioners and Dental Care Professionals in General Dental Practice*. Resuscitation Council (UK), London.

Tunstall-Pedoe H, Bailey L, Chamberlain D *et al.* (1992) Survey of 3765 cardiopulmonary resuscitations in British hospitals (the BRESUS study): methods and overall results. *BMJ*; 304:1347–1351.

Waalewijn R, de Vos R, Tijssen J, Koster R (2001) Survival models for out-of-hospital cardiopulmonary resuscitation from the perspectives of the bystander, the first responder and the paramedic. *Resuscitation*; 51:113–122.

Wrenn K (1990) The hazards of defibrillation through nitroglycerin patches. *Annals of Emergency Medicine*; 19:1327–1328.

AUTOMATED EXTERNAL
DEFIBRILLATION

Chapter 12
Paediatric emergencies

INTRODUCTION

Paediatric emergencies in the dental practice are fortunately very rare. However, if an emergency occurs, it is important to be able to respond quickly, effectively and safely. A sick child can deteriorate rapidly; it is most important to promptly recognise that a child is ill (ABCDE approach) and ensure appropriate help is sought. This may involve contacting the GP or calling 999 for an ambulance, depending on the situation. It is also important not to forget the child's parents or carer as they will usually be very upset and anxious.

If the child has a cardiopulmonary arrest in the dental practice, the adult resuscitation guidelines can be followed with just a few modifications to make them more suitable for a child. Cardiopulmonary arrest will most likely be secondary to a problem either with the airway or with breathing; hence the initial importance of oxygenation and ventilation.

To avoid misunderstanding, in this chapter, the terms 'child' and 'children' refer to both infants and children; when infants and children are specifically referred to, an infant can be defined as less than 1 year and a child from 1 year to puberty.

The aim of this chapter is to provide a brief overview to the management of paediatric emergencies.

LEARNING OUTCOMES

At the end of this chapter the reader will be able to:

- Outline the ABCDE assessment of a sick child
- Discuss the principles of paediatric resuscitation
- Describe the procedure for placing a child into the recovery position
- Discuss the management of foreign body airway obstruction

Basic Guide to Medical Emergencies in the Dental Practice, Second Edition. Phil Jevon.
© 2014 John Wiley & Sons, Ltd. Published 2014 by John Wiley & Sons, Ltd.
Companion website: www.wiley.com\go\jevon\medicalemergencies

> ## Age definitions for infants and children
>
> *Infant* < 1 year
>
> *Child* 1 year to puberty (use common sense)
>
> (Resuscitation Council (UK), 2011)

ABCDE ASSESSMENT OF A SICK CHILD

The ABCDE assessment of the sick patient has been described in detail in Chapter 3. The same approach can be adopted when assessing a child, but with some modifications and additional considerations.

Whenever possible, keep the parent with the child when undertaking the assessment. Taking the child away from the parent may cause distress. If it is necessary to administer oxygen, ideally use a paediatric non-rebreathe mask (Figure 12.1); if the child does not tolerate this, asking the parent to hold an oxygen source near the child's face may be helpful.

Airway

Asking an infant or small child to talk in order to confirm airway patency will not be appropriate – look for other indicators of airway patency, e.g. vocalising and crying (Resuscitation Council (UK), 2011).

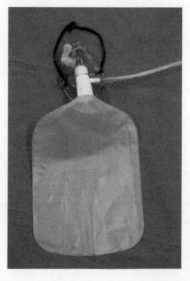

Figure 12.1 Paediatric non-rebreathe mask.

PAEDIATRIC EMERGENCIES

Breathing

Normal respiratory rates are higher in children:

- <1 year: 30–40 breaths per minute;
- 1–2 years: 26–34 breaths per minute;
- 2–5 years: 24–30 breaths per minute;
- 5–12 years 20–24 breaths per minute;
- >12 years: 12–20 breaths per minute.

Source: Resuscitation Council (UK) (2011)

Look for chest recession or retractions (sternal, subcostal or intercostals) (indication of respiratory distress) (Resuscitation Council (UK), 2011).

Circulation

Normal pulse rates are higher in infants and children who are awake:

- 3 months–2 years: 100–180 beats per minute;
- 2–10 years: 60–140 beats per minute;
- >10 years: 60–100 beats per minute.

Source: Resuscitation Council (UK) (2011)

Disability

Assess the child's interaction with his parents and surroundings. The parents will probably be able to advise whether this interaction is normal or not. Assess posture and tone: a seriously ill child becomes floppy.

Exposure

In any child who is unwell, look for the presence of tiny pin prick spots that can develop into purple bruising (purpuric rash) (Meningitis UK, 2013). This suggests bacterial meningitis. Try the tumbler test: press a glass tumbler against the rash – the rash will be visible through the glass and does not fade (Figure 12.2).

If exposing a child, take appropriate measures to minimise heat loss (particularly in infants) and respect the child's dignity (Resuscitation Council (UK), 2011).

If possible record a core temperature, particularly if pyrexia is suspected.

PRINCIPLES OF PAEDIATRIC RESUSCITATION

When undertaking paediatric resuscitation, the adult resuscitation guidelines described in Chapter 9 can be followed, with some minor modifications (Resuscitation Council (UK), 2013). In this section, the modifications are

(sidebar: PAEDIATRIC EMERGENCIES)

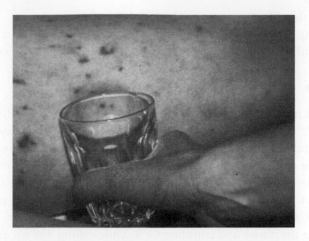

Figure 12.2 Suspected bacterial meningitis: the tumbler test. *Source:* Meningitis Research Foundation, Registered Charity 1091105. Reproduced with permission.

listed, together with some background information, which the reader may find helpful.

Priorities

The two key priorities of resuscitation in children are:

- *Oxygenation and ventilation:* cardiorespiratory arrest in children is usually due to hypoxia (low oxygen levels in the blood);
- *Effective basic life support:* the most common cardiac arrhythmia is profound bradycardia (very slow heart rate) deteriorating to asystole (therefore, the defibrillator is not usually required) (Resuscitation Council (UK), 2011).

Therefore, the adult sequence of resuscitation described in Chapter 9 would not be ideal if it was followed when resuscitating a child. However, a few minor modifications would make it suitable.

Modifications to the adult resuscitation guidelines

The procedure for resuscitation in children can follow the adult resuscitation guidelines; however, four minor modifications will make the sequence more suitable for use in children (Resuscitation Council (UK), 2011; Jevon, 2012):

- Administer five initial ventilations before starting chest compressions.
- If alone, perform CPR for 1 minute before calling 999 for an ambulance.

PAEDIATRIC EMERGENCIES

- Compress the chest approximately one-third of its depth.
- Use two fingers when compressing the chest in an infant and in a child use one or two hands as needed to achieve the recommended depth of compression.

When to call 999 for an ambulance

As soon as it is confirmed that the child is not breathing normally, send someone to call 999 for an ambulance immediately. It is an emergency situation.

If the dental practitioner is alone (extremely rare), it is recommended to perform CPR for approximately 1 minute first before calling 999 (even if she has a mobile phone) (Resuscitation Council (UK), 2011). The rationale for this is that prompt effective CPR may actually revive the child. It may be possible, after performing CPR for approximately 1 minute, to actually carry an infant or small child to the phone and continue CPR while calling 999 for an ambulance; this is recommended by some authorities (St John Ambulance *et al.*, 2011).

Airway management

The airway in an unconscious child can easily become obstructed by a combination of flexion of the neck, relaxation of the jaw, displacement of the tongue against the posterior wall of the pharynx and collapse of the hypopharynx; sometimes just opening the airway may revive the child (Jevon, 2009).

The airway can be opened by tilting the head and lifting the chin; this will help to open the airway and bring the tongue forward from the posterior wall of the pharynx (the tongue is the most common cause of airway obstruction in an unconscious child; Jevon, 2012). The neutral position in an infant (Figure 12.3) and sniffing the morning air position in a child (Figure 12.4) are recommended (Resuscitation Council (UK), 2011).

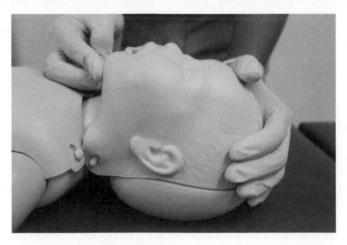

Figure 12.3 Opening the airway in an infant.

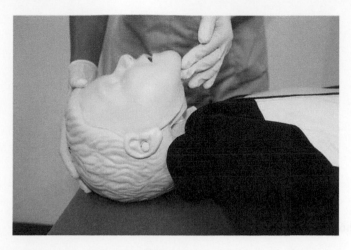

Figure 12.4 Opening the airway in a child.

Care should be taken not to press on the soft tissues under the chin as this may obstruct the airway, and blind finger sweeps are not recommended (Resuscitation Council (UK), 2011). As in adults, if there is a history of trauma, the jaw thrust rather than head tilt/chin lift is recommended (Resuscitation Council (UK), 2011).

An oropharyngeal airway can be used if there is difficulty achieving a patent airway, though particular care should be exercised if inserting one.

Ventilations

Once it is established that the child is not breathing normally, administer five initial ventilations (Figure 12.5) before, if needed, starting chest compressions at a ratio

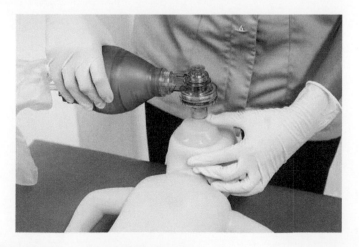

Figure 12.5 Ventilations using a self-inflating bag.

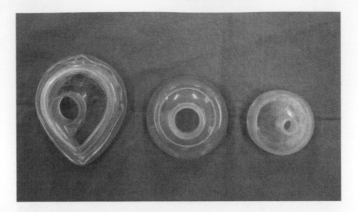

Figure 12.6 Paediatric face masks.

of 30 compressions to 2 ventilations (Resuscitation Council (UK), 2011). While performing these ventilations, send a colleague to call 999 for an ambulance.

It is recommended that a variety of child face masks (Figure 12.6) for attaching to a self-inflating bag should be immediately available in the dental practice (Resuscitation Council (UK), 2011). Ideally, a paediatric self-inflating bag should also be available, though in practice most dental practices will only have an adult bag available. An adult self-inflating bag can be used, though care should be taken to ensure that it is only squeezed enough to achieve visible chest rise. Regardless of the bag used, attach high flow oxygen (15 l/min) as soon as possible.

The use of a pocket mask is another option. The standard adult pocket mask can be used in an infant: position it upside down on the infant's face, ensuring that it covers the eye sockets as well as the nose and mouth (i.e. to achieve an effective seal) (Figure 12.7). A paediatric pocket mask is also available (Figure 12.8).

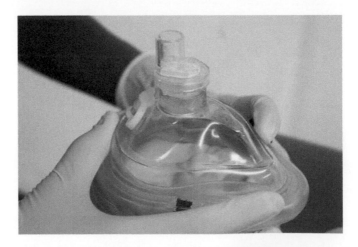

Figure 12.7 Using an adult pocket mask in an infant (upside down).

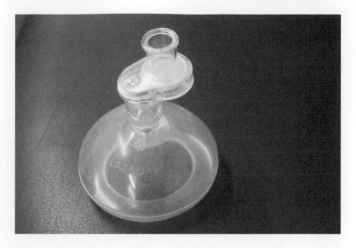

Figure 12.8 Paediatric pocket mask.

If performing mouth-to-mouth resuscitation, apply a barrier face shield if one is available and if trained to use it. The principles of mouth-to-mouth ventilation in adults have been discussed in detail in Chapter 10 ('Mouth-to-mouth ventilation'). If performing mouth-to-mouth ventilation in an infant, place your mouth over the infant's nose and mouth to deliver the ventilations; in a child the technique used in adults can be followed. NB: just inflate sufficient air to achieve chest rise. After the initial five ventilations, perform 30 chest compressions to two ventilations as described above.

Chest compressions

The principles of performing chest compressions in children are the same as in adults, with two minor modifications:

- Compress the chest approximately one-third of its depth.
- Use two fingers when compressing the chest in an infant and in a child use one or two hands as needed to achieve the recommended depth of compression.

Chest compressions in an infant
- Deliver five initial ventilations.
- Place the tips of two fingers in the centre of the chest (taking care not to press on the lower tip of the sternum, the ribs or the abdomen) (Figure 12.9).
- Compress the chest vertically down about one-third of its depth and then release the pressure to allow the chest to fully re-expand (without losing contact with the chest) (St John Ambulance *et al.*, 2011). Not allowing the chest to fully re-expand will hinder venous return to the heart and reduce the blood flow to the vital organs (Jevon, 2012).

PAEDIATRIC EMERGENCIES

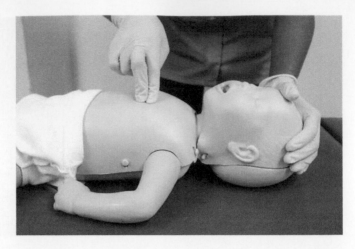

Figure 12.9 Chest compressions in an infant.

- Compress the chest at a rate of 100–120 beats per minute with a ratio of 30 compressions to 2 ventilations (Resuscitation Council (UK), 2011).
- If alone, after performing CPR for approximately 1 minute, call 999 for an ambulance.

Chest compressions in a child

- Deliver five initial ventilations.
- Place the heal of one hand in the centre of the chest (taking care not to press on the lower tip of the sternum, the ribs or the abdomen) (Figure 12.10a). In an older child or if struggling to achieve the recommended compression depth, use the two-handed technique (Figure 12.10b).
- Compress the chest vertically down about one-third of its depth and then release the pressure to allow the chest to fully re-expand (without losing contact with the chest) (St John Ambulance *et al.*, 2011).
- Compress the chest at a rate of 100–120 beats per minute with a ratio of 30 compressions to 2 ventilations (Resuscitation Council (UK), 2011).
- If working alone, after performing CPR for approximately 1 minute, call 999 for an ambulance.

The use of automated external defibrillators in children

Most cardiac arrests in children are secondary to a life-threatening airway or breathing problem; as discussed above, the initial priorities in paediatric resuscitation are to open and clear the airway and ventilate with high-concentration oxygen; defibrillation is rarely indicated.

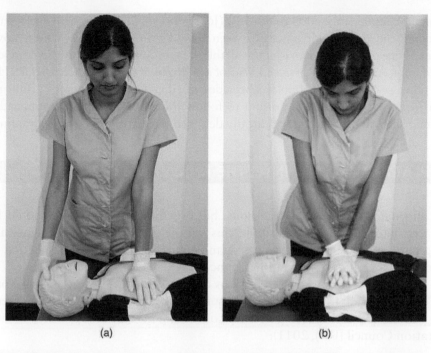

(a)   (b)

Figure 12.10 Chest compressions in a child: **(a)** one-handed technique; **(b)** two-handed technique.

However, very occasionally the primary cause of a paediatric cardiorespiratory arrest will be ventricular fibrillation (see Chapter 11), a shockable rhythm. Automated external defibrillators (AEDs) have been used successfully in children (Gurnett and Atkins, 2000; Konig *et al.*, 2005). Most AED manufacturers now supply paediatric pads (Figure 12.11) or programmes that will usually limit the

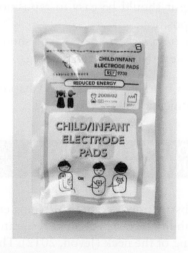

Figure 12.11 Paediatric AED pads.

PAEDIATRIC EMERGENCIES

voltage output of the AED to 50–75 J (Jorgenson *et al.*, 2002); these devices are recommended for children aged between 1 and 8 years (Berg *et al.*, 2004). However, if one of these devices is not available, it is recommended to use an unmodified adult AED in children over 1 year of age (Resuscitation Council (UK), 2011).

The use of AEDs in adults has been described in detail in Chapter 11. If using an AED in a child, it is important to follow the manufacturer's recommendations, particularly if using specifically designed paediatric pads or programme.

PLACING A CHILD INTO THE RECOVERY POSITION

If an infant or child is unconscious, but breathing normally, she should be placed into the recovery position; this will help to prevent the tongue falling back and obstructing the airway and will reduce the risk of inhalation of stomach contents (Resuscitation Council (UK), 2011).

There are several recovery positions currently advocated, but no single one can be endorsed. However, there are some important key principles that need to be followed when placing an infant or child in the recovery position (Resuscitation Council (UK), 2011):

- *Lateral position:* as far as possible, the true lateral position should be adopted, with the mouth dependent to allow free drainage of fluid.
- *Stability:* the position used should be stable; in an infant a rolled-up cushion or blanket (or similar) placed behind the back may be necessary to maintain the position.
- *Ease of monitoring:* it should be possible to easily observe (and access) the airway and monitor breathing.
- *Ease of repositioning:* it should be easy to reposition the child or roll her back into the supine position.
- *Avoidance of pressure on the chest:* the position should not result in pressure being applied to the chest that impairs breathing.

The recovery position in adults described in Chapter 7 can be used in children, though some modification may be required.

MANAGEMENT OF FOREIGN BODY AIRWAY OBSTRUCTION

Foreign body airway obstruction is a life-threatening emergency, often characterised by a sudden inability to talk, maximal respiratory effort, development of cyanosis and clutching of the neck (Jevon, 2012). There may be a history of the child eating a sweet or playing with a small object.

PAEDIATRIC EMERGENCIES

Back slaps, chest thrusts and abdominal thrusts can all help expel a foreign body from the airway (Resuscitation Council (UK), 2011); however, in 50% of choking episodes, more than one technique will be required to relieve the obstruction (Redding, 1979).

Blind finger sweeps

In all situations it would be helpful to remove any obvious foreign body from the mouth, but blind finger sweeps are not recommended as they could further impact the foreign body (Jevon, 2012) and may actually cause pharyngeal trauma.

Resuscitation Council (UK) choking guidelines

The Resuscitation Council (UK) adult choking guidelines (see Chapter 10) are also suitable for use in children over 1 year of age. They can also be followed for an infant, but with a slight modification, i.e. chest thrusts instead of abdominal thrusts (Resuscitation Council (UK), 2011).

Effective and ineffective cough

In a conscious child the treatment is determined by whether he has an effective cough or not (Resuscitation Council (UK), 2011):

- *Effective cough:* crying or a verbal response to questions, loud cough, ability to breathe before coughing and fully responsive;
- *Ineffective cough:* inability to vocalise, quiet or silent cough, inability to breathe, cyanosis and decreasing level of consciousness.

Treatment of an infant with foreign body airway obstruction

If the infant has foreign body airway obstruction, but has an effective cough, encourage him/her to cough. If the infant has (or is developing) an ineffective cough, but is still conscious (Resuscitation Council (UK), 2011; Jevon, 2012):

1. Call out for help.
2. Support the infant in a prone position, e.g. resting on your forearm or across your lap, ensuring that the head is lower than the chest (gravity will assist removal of the foreign body) and the head is well supported.
3. Deliver up to five sharp blows between the shoulder blades using the heel of the hand (Figure 12.12). If the back slaps fail to dislodge the foreign body, proceed to chest thrusts.
4. Turn the infant into a supine position, ensuring again that the head is lower than the chest.
5. Deliver up to five chest thrusts to the sternum (similar to chest compressions, but more vigorous, sharper and slower, at a rate of one every 3 seconds) (Jevon, 2012).

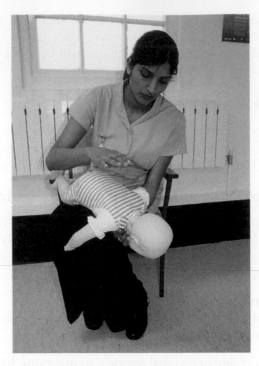

Figure 12.12 Treatment of FBAO in an infant: back blows.

6. Recheck the mouth and carefully remove any visible foreign body.
7. If the airway remains obstructed, repeat the above steps as necessary.

If the infant becomes unconscious, if not already, ask a colleague to call 999 for an ambulance and follow the resuscitation protocols, i.e. open and clear the airway, attempt to deliver five ventilations before starting chest compressions (ratio 30:2 as mentioned previously).

Abdominal thrusts are NOT recommended in infants (Resuscitation Council (UK), Resuscitation Council (UK), 2011)

Treatment of a child with foreign body airway obstruction

This is the same as for adults, as described in Chapter 10, and therefore only a brief description is required here. If the child has an ineffective cough, administer back blows (Figure 12.13); if these fail to dislodge the foreign body, proceed to abdominal thrusts.

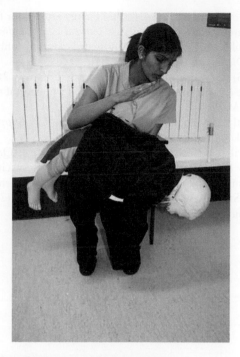

Figure 12.13 Treatment of FBAO in a child: back blows.

CONCLUSION

Paediatric emergencies in the dental practice are rare. If one occurs, it is important to be able to respond quickly, effectively and safely. In this chapter an overview has been provided of the management of paediatric emergencies. The ABCDE assessment of a sick child has been outlined and the principles of paediatric resuscitation have been discussed. The procedure for placing a child into the recovery position and the management of foreign body airway obstruction have been described.

REFERENCES

Berg R, Chapman F, Berg M *et al.* (2004) Attenuated adult biphasic shocks compared with weight-based monophasic shocks in a swine model or prolonged pediatric ventricular fibrillation. *Resuscitation*; 61:189–197.

Gurnett C, Atkins D (2000) Successful use of a biphasic waveform automated external defibrillator in a high-risk child. *American Journal of Cardiology*; 86:1051–1053.

Jevon P (2009) *Advanced Cardiac Life Support*, 2nd edn. Wiley-Blackwell, Oxford.

Jevon P (2012) *Paediatric Advanced Life Support*, 2nd edn. Wiley-Blackwell, Oxford

Jorgenson D, Morgan C, Snyder D *et al.* (2002) Energy attenuator for pediatric application of an automated external defibrillator. *Critical Care Medicine*; 30:S145–S147.

Konig B, Benger J, Goldsworthy L (2005) Automated external defibrillation in a 6-year-old. *Archives of Disease in Childhood*; 90:310–311.

Meningitis UK (2013) www.meningitisuk.org (accessed 04 May 2013).

Redding J (1979) The choking controversy: critique of evidence of the Heimlich maneuver. *Critical Care Medicine*; 7:475–479.

Resuscitation Council (UK) (2011) *Paediatric Immediate Life Support*, 2nd edn. Resuscitation Council (UK), London.

Resuscitation Council (UK) (2013) *General Dental Practice: Quality Standards for Cardiopulmonary Resuscitation Practice and Training*. Resuscitation Council (UK), London, www.resus.org.uk (accessed 05 May 2013) (draft format).

St John Ambulance, St Andrew's Ambulance, British Red Cross (2011) *First Aid Manual*, 9th edn. Dorling Kindersley, London.

Chapter 13

An overview of emergency drugs in the dental practice

INTRODUCTION

The Resuscitation Council (UK) (2012a, 2013a) has provided guidance on what emergency drugs should be available in the dental practice to treat medical emergencies (Box 13.1). All drugs should be stored together, ideally in a purpose-designed container (Greenwood, 2009). The A4 size *Emergency Drugs in the Dental Practice* guide (Figure 13.1) is a useful aide memoire (drug doses, routes of administration, etc.) and is designed to be stored in the container containing the emergency drugs. Expiry dates of the drugs should be checked and there should be a planned replacement programme in place (Resuscitation Council (UK), 2012a).

The aim of this chapter is to understand the use of emergency drugs in the dental practice.

LEARNING OUTCOMES

At the end of the chapter the reader will be able to discuss the use of the following emergency drugs:

- Adrenaline
- Aspirin
- Glucagon
- Glyceryl trinitrate (GTN) spray
- Midazolam
- Oral glucose solution/tablets/gel/powder
- Salbutamol inhaler

> **Box 13.1   The Resuscitation Council (UK) (2012a, 2013a) guidance on what emergency drugs should be available in the dental practice to treat medical emergencies**
>
> - Adrenaline injection (1:1,000, 1 mg/ml)
> - Aspirin dispersible 300 mg
> - Glucagon injection 1 mg
> - Glyceryl trinitrate (GTN) spray (400 µg/dose)
> - Oral glucose solution/tablets/gel/powder
> - Midazolam 10 mg (buccal)
> - Salbutamol aerosol inhaler (100 µg/actuation)

ADRENALINE

Adrenaline is the most important drug in anaphylaxis (McLean-Tooke *et al.*, 2003). Although there are no randomised controlled trials supporting its use, adrenaline is a logical treatment (Brown, 2005) and there is consistent anecdotal evidence endorsing its use to ease breathing difficulty and restore adequate cardiac output (Resuscitation Council (UK), 2012a).

Mode of action

Adrenaline's alpha-receptor agonist effects reverse peripheral vasodilation and reduce oedema. Its beta-receptor agonist effects dilate the bronchial airways, increase the force of myocardial contraction and suppress histamine and leukotriene release. There are also beta-2 adrenergic receptors on mast cells (Kay and Peachell, 2005) that inhibit activation (Chong *et al.*, 1995), and so early adrenaline attenuates the severity of IgE-mediated allergic reactions (Resuscitation Council (UK), 2012b). Adrenaline seems to be most effective when administered early after the onset of the reaction (Bautista *et al.*, 2002).

Presentation

Pre-filled syringe

Where possible, adrenaline should be in a pre-filled syringe (Resuscitation Council (UK), 2012a). There are currently two products available. UCB's adrenaline 500 µg product is preferable because this is the recommended does in adults (the graduated syringe also enables use in children).

Walsall Healthcare
For One & All

EMERGENCY DRUGS IN THE DENTAL PRACTICE

Walsall Healthcare NHS
NHS Trust

Drug	Indication	Adult Dose & Route	Paediatric Dose & Route
Adrenaline 1:1000 (1 mg/ml)[2]	Anaphylaxis	500 micrograms (0.5 mls 1:1000) IM May be repeated at 5 min intervals according to BP	<6 yrs: 150 micrograms (0.15 mls 1:1000) IM 6-12 yrs: 300 micrograms (0.3 mls 1:1000) IM >12 yrs: 500 micrograms (0.5 mls 1:1000) IM
Aspirin 300 mg[1]	Suspected heart attack	300 mg oral (crushed or chewed)	N/A
Glucagon 1 mg[1,2]	Hypoglycaemia (severe) (impaired consciousness, uncooperative/unable to swallow)	1 mg IM	<8 yrs (<25 kg): 0.5 mg IM >8yrs (>25 kg): 1 mg IM
Glucose[1,2]	Hypoglycaemia	15-20 g short acting carbohydrate oral e.g glass lucozade/fruit juice, ≥glucose tablets/5 sweets or 25 g tube glucogel (10 g carbohydrate): oral or gently squeeze into cheek, rub outside of cheek to aid absorption. Repeat after 15 mins if required	Dose as for adults
Glyceryl Trinitrate Spray (400 micrograms/dose)[1]	Angina or suspected heart attack	1-2 actuations sublingually (no more than 3 doses recommended at any one time)	N/A
Midazolam[1,3]	Prolonged, acute convulsive seizures lasting ≥ 5 mins or repeated (≥3 in one hour) (NICE 2012)	10mg buccal (unlicensed for use in adults)	1 <5 yrs: 5 mg buccal* 5 <10 yrs: 7.5 mg buccal* 10 to <18 yrs: 10 mg buccal* * a buccal midazolam (in pre-filled syringes) is licensed for the treatment of prolonged, acute convulsive seizures in children up to the age of 18 yrs. Age specific doses are recommended.
Salbutamol Inhaler 100 micrograms/dose	Asthma attack	1-2 actuations inhaled Repeat if required	Dose as for adults

References
1. Resuscitation Council (UK) (2012) Medical emergencies and resuscitation-standards for clinical practice and training for dental practitioners and dental care professionals in general dental practice (revised February 2012)
2. Diabetes UK (2012) Hypoglycaemia www.diabetes.org.uk (accessed 2 June 2012)
3. NICE (2012) The epilepsies, the diagnosis and management of the epilepsies in adults and children in primary and secondary care www.nice.org.uk (accessed 2 June 2012)

Further Reading
Jevon P (2013) Medical Emergencies in the Dental Practice 2nd Edition Wiley Blackwell, Oxford
The production of this poster was made possible with an educational grant from VeriPharma Limited

WALSALL HEALTHCARE NHS TRUST DECEMBER 2012

Figure 13.1 'Emergency Drugs in the Dental Practice' guide. Source: Walsall Healthcare NHS Trust. Reproduced with permission.

Ampoules

As repeated dose of adrenaline may be required, most dental practices will also stock adrenaline 1:1000 ampoules that usually come in a box of 10. It is recommended to use a 23 g (blue) needle, or in a larger patient, a 21 g (green) needle, for the intramuscular (IM) injection (Resuscitation Council (UK), 2012b).

Auto-injector devices

Although it would be reasonable to use an auto-injector device if one is immediately available (i.e. patient's own device), they are primarily for self-use by patients who are at risk of anaphylaxis (Resuscitation Council (UK), 2012b); their routine use by dental practitioners is not recommended because:

* Auto-injectors are relatively expensive with a limited shelf life compared with the cost of an ampoule of adrenaline and syringe and needle;
* Anaphylactic reactions are rare and most auto-injectors purchased for dental practices will not be used;
* Auto-injectors come with standard length of needle which may not be long enough to administer IM adrenaline for some patients;
* Most healthcare staff likely to deal with an anaphylactic reaction in the healthcare setting should have the skills to draw up adrenaline and administer IM injection of adrenaline.

Source: Resuscitation Council (UK) (2013b)

Indication

Anaphylaxis.

Dose and route of administration

* 500 µg (0.5 ml 1:1000) IM.
* The dose is repeated if necessary at 5 minute intervals according to blood pressure, pulse and respiratory function (Resuscitation Council (UK), 2012a).

Paediatric doses
* <6 years: 150 µg (0.15 ml 1:1000) IM.
* 6–12 years: 300 µg (0.3 ml 1:1000) IM.
* >12 years: 500 µg (0.5 ml 1:1000) IM.

Side effects

Side effects include palpitations, dry mouth and tremor. The only reported severe adverse effect following intramuscular administration of adrenaline was a myocardial infarction in a patient with severe ischaemic heart disease (Saff *et al.*, 1993).

ASPIRIN

Aspirin is recommended in a suspected heart attack for its anti-platelet effect. The benefits of administering aspirin are well known. It halves the rate of vascular events (cardiovascular death, non-fatal myocardial infarction and non-fatal stroke) in patients with unstable angina and reduces it by nearly a third in those with acute myocardial infarction (heart attack) (Fox *et al.*, 2004).

Mode of action

Aspirin depletes platelet aggregation and inhibit thrombus formation in the arterial circulation because in faster-flowing blood vessels thrombi are composed mainly of platelets and little fibrin

Presentation

Soluble aspirin 300 mg. It is sometimes stored in a 'child-proof' container, in which case it will be necessary to 'marry-up' the arrows before it is possible to open the container.

Indication

Suspected heart attack.

Dose and route of administration

• 300 mg crushed or chewed.

Paediatric doses

Not recommended for use in children.

Side effects

Anaphylactic reaction.

Contra-indications

Known allergy to aspirin (NICE, 2012).

GLUCAGON

Glucagon, a polypeptide hormone produced by the alpha cells of the islets of Langerhans in the pancreas, mobilises glycogen (stored glucose) stores in the liver thus increasing the patient's blood sugar levels. After administration, once the patient is alert and able to swallow, he should be offered a drink containing glucose and if possible some food high in carbohydrate (Resuscitation Council (UK), 2012a).

Mode of action

Glucagon increases the patient's blood sugar levels by mobilising glycogen in the liver. It should be effective within 10 minutes (Novo Nordisk Ltd, 2013). Glucagon may be ineffective if the patient:

• has been fasting for a long time;
• has low levels of adrenaline;
• is suffering from chronic hypoglycaemia;
• has alcohol-induced hypoglycaemia;
• has a tumour that releases glucagon or insulin.

Source: Novo Nordisk Ltd (2013)

Presentation

Glucagon injection is available as GlucaGen® Hypokit. This comes in an orange tamper-evident container which contains glucagon powder for re-constitution and a syringe with a pre-filled syringe containing water for injection.

GlucaGen can be stored either in a refrigerator (2°C–8°C), or out of a refrigerator below 25°C for up to 18 months within the shelf-life period (Novo Nordisk Ltd, 2013). The advantage of storing GlucaGen with the dental practice's other emergency drugs is that it keeps all the drugs together in one place. It should be stored in the original package (orange container) to protect from light.

Indications

Confirmed or suspected hypoglycaemia when oral glucose cannot be administered orally, or if the patient is unconscious.

Dose and route of administration

1 MG IM (Resuscitation Council UK, 2012a)

Paediatric doses
- Children > 25 kg (>6–8 years): 1 mg IM.
- Children < 25 kg (<6–8 years): 0.5 mg IM.

Source: Novo Nordisk Ltd (2013)

Side effects

Side effects are rare but can include nausea, vomiting and abdominal pain.

GLYCERYL TRINITRATE SPRAY

Glyceryl trinitrate (GTN) is rapidly absorbed through the buccal and sub-lingual mucosa, and in human, peak concentrations in plasma are observed within 4 minutes of sublingual administration (MHRA, 2013).

Mode of action

GTN acts on vascular smooth muscles to produce arterial and venous vasodil-atation that results in a reduction of venous return and an improvement in myocardial perfusion (blood flow to the muscle of the heart) with the result of a reduction in the work performed by the heart and hence reduced oxygen demand (MHRA, 2013).

Indications

- Angina (patient with known coronary heart disease) (see later);
- Suspected heart attack.

Patients with known coronary heart disease should be given clear advice on how to self-medicate with GTN to relieve the symptoms of their angina.

- An initial dose should be taken at symptom onset.
- If necessary, a further two doses should be taken at 5 minute intervals.
- If symptoms have not settled within 5 minutes of taking the third dose (15 minutes in total from onset of symptoms) emergency medical services should be contacted.

Source: SIGN (2013)

Presentation

GTN spray typically comes in an aluminium pressurised container, sealed with a metered spray valve, providing 200 metered doses of 400 µg. Although GTN can also be administered in tablet format, most dental practices stock the spray as recommended by the Resuscitation Council (UK), 2012a).

Dose and route of administration

One or two metered doses (400–800 µg) GTN be sprayed under the tongue while the patient holds his breath. No more than three doses are recommended at any one time.

The dose may be repeated.

Paediatric doses

GTN spray is not recommended in children.

Side effects

Side effects include headache, palpitations and hypotension (low blood pressure).

MIDAZOLAM

The British National Formulary, Advanced Paediatric Life Support course, national epilepsy organisations and Royal College of Paediatrics and Child Health have, for a number of years, recommended buccal midazolam for the emergency treatment of prolonged convulsive seizures (Resuscitation Council (UK), 2012c). Until recently no licensed formulation was available and unlicensed 'specials' were used. Buccolam® is now available that has a license for use in less than 18 years of age.

Buccolam®

Buccolam (midazolam oromucosal solution) has recently acquired a paediatric use marketing authorisation (PUMA) from the European Commission (European Medicines Agency, 2011) to become the first and only licensed oromucosal midazolam for the treatment of prolonged, acute, convulsive seizures in infants, children and adolescents (from 3 months to <18 years of age) (Jevon, 2012a, 2012b). Following buccal administration, it is rapidly absorbed across the mucous membranes directly into the bloodstream. Clinical studies show that cessation of visible signs of seizures within 10 minutes was achieved in 65–78% of children receiving oromucosal midazolam (Jevon, 2012a, 2012b).

Its use in adults remains 'off label' but the Resuscitation Council (UK) (2012c) recommends a 10 mg (2 ml) dose for adults (as for the older child) and considers that such 'off label' use of a licensed product is justified in the emergency situation (Resuscitation Council (UK), 2012c).

In both 'licensed' and 'off label' settings, the drug does not need to have been prescribed to the patient when used in an emergency but in the dental practice, it should, however, be administered by (or under the supervision of) a dental practitioner (Resuscitation Council (UK), 2012c).

Reclassification of midazolam as a Schedule 3 Controlled Drug

Concerns have been raised regarding the recent reclassification of midazolam as a 'Schedule 3' Controlled Drug. Although this reclassification does require certain legal processes, there is no legal requirement for midazolam to be stored in a locked cupboard or to maintain a midazolam-controlled drug register (Resuscitation Council (UK), 2012b).

Ordering stocks of midazolam

Concerns have also been raised regarding the ordering of stocks of midazolam for use in the emergency treatment of seizures. A dentist can issue a requisition for any licensed product for use within their practice, as appropriate, using the standardised requisition form: FP10CDF (Resuscitation Council (UK), 2012c).

Dentists who do not use midazolam on a regular basis can still requisite this Schedule 3 Drug under the conditions laid out by the Royal Pharmaceutical Society of Great Britain in their guidance 'Medicines, Ethics and Practice: the professional guide for pharmacists' (Resuscitation Council (UK), 2012c).

Mode of action

Midazolam belongs to a group of medicines called benzodiazepines that have a sedative action.

Presentation

- Buccolam is available in age-specific, pre-filled, plastic, oral syringes and has a shelf life of 18 months. It is available as a 5 mg/ml solution for use in children up to 18 years.
- Midazolam injection solution 10 mg/2 ml ampoules (unlicensed) (British Medical Association and the Royal Pharmaceutical Society of Great Britain, 2013).

(Other unlicensed formulations are available which may have different doses – refer to the product literature.)

Source: British Medical Association and the Royal Pharmaceutical Society of Great Britain (2013)

Indications

The National Institute for Health and Clinical Excellence (NICE) has recently published updated guidance on the management of prolonged convulsive seizures, recommending the administration of buccal midazolam as first-line treatment in children and adults with prolonged (>5 minutes) or repeated (more than three in an hour) seizures in the community (NICE, 2012). The Resuscitation Council (UK) has endorsed this (Resuscitation Council (UK), 2012a).

Dose and route of administration

- 10 mg via buccal route.

Procedure for administering Buccolam

- Select appropriate age-specific dose for the patient.
- Remove the syringe cap (do not attach a needle to the syringe: Buccolam must not be injected).
- Carefully and slowly advance the syringe into the space between the gum and the cheek and insert the Buccolam liquid (for larger volumes of Buccolam and/or smaller patients, it is recommended to insert slowly half the volume into one side of the mouth and then the other half into the other side).

Source: Viropharma, 2013

Procedure for administering midazolam injection

If midazolam injection is administered (unlicensed), then the needle must be removed from the syringe before the midazolam is squirted into the buccal cavity.

Paediatric doses

- Child 1–5 years: 5 mg.
- Child 5–10 years: 7.5 mg.
- Child above 10 years: 10 mg.

Source: Resuscitation Council (UK) (2012a)

Side effects

Side effects include drowsiness and respiratory depression.

AN OVERVIEW OF EMERGENCY DRUGS IN THE DENTAL PRACTICE

ORAL GLUCOSE SOLUTION/TABLETS/GEL/POWDER

Where the patient is co-operative and conscious with an intact gag reflex, 10–20 g of fast acting glucose should be offered (may need to be repeated in 10–15 minutes) (Resuscitation Council (UK), 2012a).

Presentation

There are many practical options for fast acting glucose (see later). Glucogel, a fast acting gel that is quickly absorbed, is also an option. Each 40% dextrose tube contains 10 g of fast acting glucose – guidelines recommend 10–20 g of fast acting glucose for the treatment of mild-to-moderate hypoglycaemia. To use it, simply twist off the cap, squeeze the contents of the whole tube into the mouth and swallow (alternatively it can be squeezed inside the patient's cheek and the outside rubbed gently to aid absorption. It is not recommended to administer glucogel to an unconscious person. Glucogel is also available in a 40% glucose 80 g bottle.

Indication

Hypoglycaemia (confirmed or suspected) where the patient is co-operative and conscious with an intact gag reflex.

Dose and route of administration

Immediately treat with 10–20 g of a fast acting glucose such as:

- a glass of non-diet soft drink such as cola or lemonade;
- three or more glucose tablets;
- five sweets, e.g. jelly babies;
- a glass or carton of fruit juice;
- glucogel (available on prescription if you are treated with insulin).

Source: Diabetes UK (2013)

SALBUTAMOL INHALER

Salbutamol (ventolin) is a short-acting beta-2 adrenergic stimulant, used in the treatment of bronchial asthma and other forms of reversible airway-obstructive diseases. Following inhalation, it is absorbed from the bronchi in the lungs.

A salbutamol inhaler is a device for the administration of inhalation of salbutamol. Various inhaler devices and formulations have been developed to help ensure the efficient and simple delivery of medications, with minimal side effects (Rees and Kanabar, 2006). *Pressurized metered dose inhalers* (pMDIs) (see Chapter 4) are the commonest type of inhaler used. They are small, convenient, easy to carry and deliver a wide range of medications (Newell and Hume, 2006). This type of inhaler is the commonest device stocked in dental practices. See Box 13.2.

Even when used properly, only 10% of the drug reaches the airways below the larynx; 50% is deposited in the mouth with close to 90% eventually being swallowed (Currie and Douglas, 2007).

Some patients, particularly children and the elderly, can find it difficult to perfect the correct technique for using a pMDI because it requires co-ordinating actuation and inhalation efficiently, and to inhale at the correct inspiratory flow rate (British Medical Association and Royal Pharmaceutical Society of Great Britain, 2013). The use of a large volume spacer device can be helpful in these patients (see Chapter 4).

Mode of action

Beta-2 adrenergic agonists act on bronchial smooth muscle inducing bronchodilation and relieving bronchospasm in asthma and chronic obstructive pulmonary disease with asthmatic features.

Asthma UK's website contains detailed advice and video clips on how to correctly use inhalers that the reader may find helpful: www.asthma.org.uk

---

Box 13.2   Suggested procedure for using a salbutamol inhaler

- Explain the procedure to the patient
- Remove the mouthpiece cover from the inhaler
- Advise the patient to shake the inhaler and then breathe out
- Advise the patient to place the mouthpiece into his mouth, then to close his lips and teeth around it
- At the start of inspiration, advise the patient to press the canister down while he continue to breathe in slowly and deeply
- Advise the patient to remove the mouthpiece from his mouth and then to close his lips
- Advise the patient to hold his breath for up to 10 seconds and then to breathe out normally
- If a second dose is required, wait 30 seconds and repeat the above steps before replacing the cover

Source: Asthma UK (2013).

Side effects

Side effects include palpitations and tremor.

Dose

Initially two activations (100 µg/actuation).

CONCLUSION

Guidance has been provided on what emergency drugs should be available in the dental practice to treat medical emergencies. In this chapter each drug has been discussed including indications, recommended doses and routes of administration. Dental practitioners must check the expiry dates of the drugs on a regular basis and there should be a planned replacement programme in place.

REFERENCES

Asthma UK (2013) www.asthma.org.uk (accessed 16 May 2013).

Bautista E, Simons F, Simons K *et al.* (2002) Epinephrine fails to hasten hemodynamic recovery in fully developed canine anaphylactic shock. *International Archives of Allergy and Immunology*; 128(2):151–164.

British Medical Association and the Royal Pharmaceutical Society of Great Britain (2013) *British National Formulary 65*. Royal Pharmaceutical Society, London.

Brown SG (2005) Cardiovascular aspects of anaphylaxis: implications for treatment and diagnosis. *Current Opinion in Allergy and Clinical Immunology*; 5(4):359–364.

Chong LK, Morice AH, Yeo WW, *et al.* (1995) Functional desensitization of beta agonist responses in human lung mast cells. *American Journal of Respiratory Cell and Molecular Biology* ; 13(5):540–546.

Currie G, Douglas J (2007) Oxygen and inhalers. In: Currie G (ed.) *ABC of COPD*, Blackwell Publishing, Oxford.

Diabetes UK (2013) www.diabetes.org.uk (accessed 14 June 2013).

European Medicines Agency (EMA) (2011) *Assessment report: Buccolam*, www.ema. europa.eu (accessed 2 June 2012).

Fox K, Mehta S, Peters R *et al.* (2004) Benefits and risks of the combination of clopidogrel land aspirin in patients undergoing surgical revascularization for non-ST-elevation acute coronary syndrome: the clopidogrel in unstable angina to prevent recurrent ischemic events (CURE) trial. *Circulation*; 110(10):1202–1208.

Greenwood M (2009) Medical emergencies in dental practice: 1. The drug box, equipment and general approach. *Dental Update*; 36:202–211.

Jevon P (2012a) Updated guidance on medical emergencies and resuscitation in the dental practice. *British Dental Journal*; 212(1): 41–43.

Jevon P (2012b) Buccolam® (buccal midazolam): a review of its use for the treatment of prolonged acute convulsive seizures in the dental practice. *British Dental Journal*; 213(2): 81–82.

Kay LJ, Peachell PT. (2005) Mast cell beta2-adrenoceptors. *Chemical Immunology and Allergy*; 87:145–153.

McLean-Tooke AP, Bethune CA, Fay AC, Spickett GP. (2003) Adrenaline in the treatment of anaphylaxis: what is the evidence? *British Medical Journal*; 327(7427):1332–1335.

MHRA (2013) *Glyceryl Trinitrate Spray 400 Micrograms per Metered Dose Sublingual Spray PL 16431/0023*, www.mhra.gov.uk (accessed 04 October 2103).

Newell K, Hume S (2006) Choosing the right inhaler for patients with asthma. *Nursing Standard*; 21(5):46–48.

NICE (2012) *The Epilepsies: The Diagnosis and Management of the Epilepsies in Adults and Children in Primary and Secondary Care*, www.nice.org.uk/cg137 (accessed 2 June 2012).

Novo Nordisk Limited (2013) www.novonordisk.co.uk (accessed 16 May 2013).

Rees J, Kanabar D (2006) *ABC of Asthma*, 5th edn. Blackwell Publishing, Oxford

Resuscitation Council (UK) (2012a) *Medical Emergencies and Resuscitation – Standards for Clinical Practice and Training for Dental Practitioners and Dental Care Professionals in General Dental Practice*, www.resus.org.uk (accessed 16 May 2013).

Resuscitation Council (UK) (2012b) *Emergency Treatment of Anaphylactic Reactions*, www.resus.org.uk (accessed 16 May 2013).

Resuscitation Council (UK) (2012c) *Emergency Use of Buccal Midazolam in Dental Practice*, www.resus.org.uk (accessed 16 May 2013).

Resuscitation Council (UK) (2013a) *General Dental Practice: Quality Standards for Cardiopulmonary Resuscitation Practice and Training* (Resuscitation Council (UK), London), www.resus.org.uk (accessed 05 May 2013) (draft format).

Resuscitation Council (UK) (2013b) *Frequently Asked Questions on Anaphylactic Reactions* (Resuscitation Council UK, London), www.resus.org.uk (accessed 05 May 2013).

Saff R, Nahhas A, Fink J (1993) Myocardial infarction induced by coronary vasospasm after self-administration of epinephrine. *Annals of Allergy*; 70:396–398.

SIGN (2013) SIGN 93: *Acute Coronary Syndromes: A National Clinical Guideline*, (accessed 06 May 2013).

Viropharma (2013) www.buccolam.co.uk (accessed 13 June 2013).

AN OVERVIEW OF EMERGENCY DRUGS IN THE DENTAL PRACTICE

Chapter 14

Principles of first aid in the dental practice

INTRODUCTION

First aid can be defined as the initial assistance or treatment given to someone who is injured or suddenly taken ill (St John Ambulance *et al.*, 2011). It can cover a wide range of scenarios ranging from simple reassurance following a minor mishap to dealing with a life-threatening emergency (Jevon, 2004).

Providing first aid can be stressful; the stress of working in unfamiliar circumstances, sometimes with inquisitive and intrusive onlookers should not be underestimated. It is important to remain calm and focussed on the priorities.

The aim of this chapter is to provide an overview to the principles of first aid in the dental practice. Some aspects of first aid, e.g. CPR, will be discussed in other parts of this book.

LEARNING OUTCOMES

At the end of the chapter the reader will be able to:

- List the priorities of first aid
- Discuss the responsibilities when providing first aid
- Outline the assessment of the casualty
- Describe the environmental hazards that may be encountered
- Discuss the treatment of wounds and severe bleeding
- Outline the treatment for minor burns and scalds
- Discuss the treatment for poisoning, stings and bites
- Discuss the importance of record keeping

Basic Guide to Medical Emergencies in the Dental Practice, Second Edition. Phil Jevon.
© 2014 John Wiley & Sons, Ltd. Published 2014 by John Wiley & Sons, Ltd.
Companion website: www.wiley.com\go\jevon\medicalemergencies

PRIORITIES OF FIRST AID

The priorities of first aid are to:

- ensure appropriate help is called if necessary;
- ensure both the rescuer's and casualty's safety;
- keep the casualty alive: i.e. particular attention to airway, breathing and circulation;
- prevent the casualty from deteriorating;
- promote the recovery of the casualty;
- provide reassurance and comfort to the casualty.

Source: Jevon (2004)

RESPONSIBILITIES WHEN PROVIDING FIRST AID

The provision of first aid is not an exact science and it is important to remember the golden rule: 'first do no harm' while applying the term 'calculated risk' (St John Ambulance *et al.*, 2011). The dental practitioner has a number of responsibilities if he is required to provide first aid.

- Assessing the situation quickly and safely;
- Ensuring appropriate help is summoned;
- Protecting the casualty and others at the scene from possible harm;
- Identifying as far as possible the cause of the illness or the nature of the injury;
- Providing first aid within her own sphere of expertise and competence;
- Ensuring that any first aid provided follows current and up-to-date guidelines, where appropriate;
- Minimising the risk of cross-infection;
- Reporting observations/findings to those taking over the care of the casualty;
- Adhering to the GDC's Code of Conduct (2005);
- Maintaining the casualty's confidentiality following the GDC's guidelines;
- Obtaining the casualty's consent (if possible) prior to administering first aid.

Source: Jevon (2004); St John Ambulance *et al.* (2011)

ASSESSMENT OF THE CASUALTY

Safe approach

The initial priority is always to ensure if it is safe to approach the casualty. This includes ensuring that measures are taken to minimise the risk of cross-infection.

Primary survey

The priority is then to assess the casualty following the ABCDE approach (see Chapter 3) to identify any life-threatening problems and provide emergency life-support treatment as required.

Secondary survey

Once it has been established that the casualty is not out of immediate danger, a secondary survey should be undertaken (St John Ambulance *et al.*, 2011) and, depending on the situation, this could involve:

- taking a history;
- looking for external clues;
- ascertaining the mechanics of injury;
- assessing signs and symptoms;
- head-to-toe survey.

Source: Jevon (2004); St John Ambulance *et al.* (2011)

Definitive care

Depending on the scenario, definitive care could involve:

- providing advice only;
- advising the casualty to visit his GP;
- arranging transport to take the casualty to hospital;
- alerting the emergency services.

Source: Jevon (2004); St John Ambulance *et al.* (2011)

Environmental hazards that may be encountered

Environmental hazards that may be encountered in the dental practice include gas, electricity, fire and poisoning.

Gas
If there is a smell of gas or a gas leak is detected:

- Open doors and windows to disperse the gas;
- Check to see if the gas supply to an appliance has been left on, unlit or if the pilot light has gone out;
- Do not smoke, use matches or naked flames;
- Do not turn electrical switches on or off – this includes the door bell;

- Turn off the gas supply at the meter (unless it is located in a cellar);
- Contact National Grid Gas Emergencies on 0800 111 999 (24 hour line).

Source: National Grid (2013); Gas Guide (2013)

Low-voltage electricity

Injuries caused by electricity often occur in the workplace environment resulting from contact with a low-voltage domestic current, usually due to a faulty switch or appliance (St John Ambulance *et al.*, 2011). The presence of water presents additional risks. The electrical contact will need to be broken.

> **NB:** do not touch the casualty if he is still in contact with the electrical current (St John Ambulance *et al.*, 2011)

Switch off the current at the mains or meter point if it can be easily reached; otherwise, remove the plug or wrench the cable free (St John Ambulance *et al.*, 2011). If unable to reach the plug, cable or mains:

- Stand on some dry insulating material, e.g. telephone directory, wooden box.
- Using a wooden object, e.g. broom, push the casualty's limbs away from the electrical source or push the latter away from the casualty. Do not use anything metallic.
- If the casualty still remains attached to the electrical current, carefully loop some rope around his ankles and pull him away from the source.

Source: Jevon (2004); St John Ambulance *et al.* (2011)

Fire

Dental practices should have an emergency plan (Box 14.1) in place in case of fire. This will be specific to the premises and will detail the pre-planned procedures in place for use in the event of a fire. This will typically involve:

- Raising the alarm: activate the nearest fire alarm and warn people who are at risk; call the fire and rescue services.
- Assessing for danger: if the fire is small, is discovered early and a fire blanket or appropriate fire extinguisher is available, try to smother the flames; if unable to extinguish the flames within 30 seconds leave the building.
- Getting to safety: leave the building and close doors behind you; do not enter a smoke-filled room; follow fire escape route if appropriate.

  Some basic principles:

- Do not use an elevator – if the electricity fails the elevator may abruptly stop working; also the elevator shaft can act like a chimney, sucking up flames and fumes.

> ## Box 14.1   Key features (where appropriate) of an emergency plan in case of fire
>
> - Action on discovering a fire
> - Warning if there is a fire
> - Calling the fire brigade
> - Evacuation of the premises including those particularly at risk
> - Power/process isolation
> - Places of assembly and roll call
> - Liaison with emergency services
> - Identification of key escape routes
> - The firefighting equipment provided
> - Specific responsibilities in the event of a fire
> - Training required
> - Provision of information to relevant persons
>
> *Source:* London Fire Brigade (2013).

- If in a room full of smoke, remain close to the floor and if possible cover the nose and mouth with a damp cloth or towel.
- Close doors on a fire.
- Never open a door that is hot or has hot handles – suggests that a fire is raging behind it.
- If unable to find an escape route, locate a fire-free room that has a window; shut the door, open the window and call out for help and remain close to the floor; if possible block any gaps under the door.
- Even if it is dark, do not turn on the light as this may cause an explosion.

Source: Jevon (2004); St John Ambulance *et al.* (2011)

Removing the casualty's clothing

Removing the casualty's clothing can make him feel more anxious and vulnerable, so it is important only to remove the clothing if it is absolutely essential and do not forget to obtain the casualty's consent, where possible, explaining to him why it is necessary to do so and always maintain his dignity.

If it is necessary to cut a garment, try to cut along the seams of trousers or sleeves (St John Ambulance *et al.*, 2011) (easier to repair the clothing) and if the casualty has a foot or leg injury, try to remove the shoe or boot before the ankle/leg becomes swollen.

If removing an upper garment when there is an upper limb injury, remove the uninjured arm before the injured arm; encourage the casualty to support the injured arm. NB: if the casualty has sustained a possible spinal injury, e.g. fallen down a flight of stairs, do not attempt to remove the upper garment.

Secondary survey

Once it is established that the casualty is not in immediate danger, a secondary survey should be performed (St John Ambulance *et al.*, 2011). Depending on the situation, this could involve:

- taking a history;
- looking for external clues;
- ascertaining the mechanics of injury;
- assessing signs and symptoms;
- undertaking a head-to-toe survey.

Source: St John Ambulance *et al.* (2011)

History
Take a history:

- Casualty details, e.g. age, past medical history, contact address, next of kin, medications etc;
- Past medical history including any medications being taken;
- Details of injury/accident, e.g. time and how it happened, mechanics of injury (see later);
- When the casualty last had something to eat or drink.

Source: Jevon (2004)

As well as asking the casualty, also question members of staff and patients as appropriate.

External clues
Look for external clues, e.g. medications, MedicAlert bracelet and check history.

Mechanics of injury
Information related to the mechanics of injury can be helpful in some situations, e.g. if the casualty fell down a flight of stairs.

Signs and symptoms
Look for any signs and ask the casualty if he has any symptoms.

Head-to-toe survey
Undertake a head-to-toe survey where appropriate.

Vital signs
Continually monitor the casualty's vital signs as appropriate.

WOUNDS AND BLEEDING

Wounds can be classified as being either an open wound, e.g. abrasion, puncture wound, or a closed wound, e.g. bruise. Wounds and bleeding can be life threatening. When providing first aid, it is important to be able to recognise which wounds can be managed in the dental practice and which will require urgent medical attention. Wounds can be caused by a number of mechanisms; the treatment and management of wounds is often determined by the mechanism of injury (Wyatt *et al.*, 2012).

When providing first aid for wounds and bleeding, it is important to ensure that the risk of infection is minimised, both to the rescuer and the casualty. If possible, sterile gloves should be worn.

Types of wounds

Abrasion (graze)
An abrasion, commonly referred to as a graze, is a superficial injury manifesting from the ripping of skin. It can be caused by a friction burn or gravel rash. Tags of skin may be evident at one end of the abrasion, indicating the edge of skin last in contact with abrading surface (Wyatt *et al.*, 2012).

Incised wound
An incised wound is a cut caused by a sharp object, e.g. knife, broken glass. Vascular damage may occur resulting in profuse bleeding. Structural damage to tendons or nerves may be complicating factors.

Laceration
A laceration is tearing or ripping of the skin; it may be superficial or may involve deeper structures and may be caused by gagged metal or broken glass. Unlike most incised wounds, haemorrhage generally tends to be less profuse, but soft tissue damage adjacent to the laceration can be significant and the risk of infection is high (St John Ambulance *et al.*, 2011).

Puncture wound
A puncture wound is normally caused by a sharp object (Wyatt *et al.*, 2012).

Bruise
A bruise, sometimes referred to as a contusion, is caused by a blunt injury to blood vessels within the tissues, resulting in tender swelling and discolouration (Wyatt *et al.*, 2012).

The site of the bruise will change in colour as the bruise develops. At its peak the bruise will be blue/black in nature and eventually fade showing a

PRINCIPLES OF FIRST AID IN THE
DENTAL PRACTICE

yellow pigment by about day five. This manifestation is the bilirubin leaking from the damaged red blood cells and is part of the bruise's normal pathology. Extensive bruising can last for several weeks.

The normal course of a bruise is to present with significant pain and lack of power and movement. Treatment consists of a cold compress, rest and elevation.

Principles of treating wounds

Wound assessment

When assessing a wound the following should be established:

- Mechanism of injury – in particular, is internal injury likely?
- Time of injury.
- Place of injury, e.g. in the garden, i.e. tetanus risk.
- Tetanus status of the casualty.
- Location of the wound.
- Circulation problems distal to wound.
- Extent of likely damage.
- In the case of a burn/scald – surface area and depth of skin affected (see pages).
- Amount of bleeding and what type (see Three categories of bleeding section).
- Presence of foreign body.

Cleaning a wound

If necessary, wash the wound under running tap water; tap water does not contain pathogenic bacteria and is often used in A & E departments to clean acute traumatic wounds (Jevon, 2004). Dry the wound and apply a dressing (sterile if possible) if necessary.

Dressings

Applying a dressing will help to keep the wound dry and will provide some degree of protection. There are many different types of wound dressings currently available. Some important points to consider when using a dressing:

- Ensure the dressing is large enough to fit comfortably and cover the wound;
- Use a sterile dressing if possible; if not available, a clean non-fluffy dressing will suffice;
- When applying the dressing, ensure to handle it using its edges;
- Use adhesive dressing for small cuts and grazes;
- If applying plaster, always ask the casualty whether he is allergic to it.

Source: Jevon (2004); St John Ambulance *et al.* (2011)

Bandages and bandaging

Bandages can be used to secure dressings, control bleeding, immobilise and support limbs and reduce swelling (St John Ambulance *et al.*, 2011).

Cold compress

The application of a cold compress can help to reduce swelling and relieve pain. It can be particularly helpful for treating bruising and sprains. There are two methods of applying a cold press: a cold pad or an ice pack.

Cold pad

- Soak a pad (towel, flannel or similar) in cold water; then wring it out.
- Apply the pad firmly over the injury.
- Regularly re-soak the pad in cold water to keep it cold.

Source: Jevon (2004); St John Ambulance *et al.* (2011)

Ice pack

- Partly fill up a plastic bag with ice cubes and then seal it (a bag of frozen vegetables will suffice).
- Wrap it up in a dry cloth or towel.
- Apply the pad firmly over the injury.
- Replace the bag as required.

NB: do not apply ice directly onto the skin, as it may burn it.

Source: Jevon (2004); St John Ambulance *et al.* (2011)

Embedded foreign objects

Embedded foreign objects can be very painful and can cause infection. Only remove them if it is easy to do so; otherwise seek medical help. **NB:** Seek urgent medical help for embedded large foreign objects, particularly those in the chest and abdomen.

Splinter

If the casualty has a small splinter, e.g. of wood, glass or metal, it may be possible to remove it using a pair of tweezers:

- Sterilise a pair of tweezers, e.g. place in boiling water for a few seconds and then let them cool;
- Gently squeeze the skin on either side of the splinter; hopefully the splinter will then be protruding out from the skin;
- Using the tweezers, grasp the splinter and pull it out at the angle it went in;
- Carefully squeeze the wound to encourage slight bleeding to flush out any remaining dirt;
- Clean and dry the area, apply adhesive dressing if necessary.

Source: Jevon (2004); St John Ambulance *et al.* (2011)

Large embedded object

A large embedded object in a wound should be left *in situ*, as further damage may be caused, particularly if it is in the chest or abdomen (the object may have pierced a blood vessel and, while it remains in the wound, may act as a 'plug' and prevent bleeding) (St John Ambulance *et al.*, 2011). First aid treatment:

- If there is bleeding from around the embedded object, apply pressure around it; do not apply pressure to the actual object.
- Place pads of gauze around the object sufficient enough to be able to bandage over it without applying pressure on it.
- Elevate the affected limb if appropriate.
- Seek medical help.

Source: Jevon (2004); St John Ambulance *et al.* (2011)

Three categories of bleeding

There are three categories of bleeding, arterial, venous and capillary:

- Arterial bleeding: usually bright red and often of a bounding pulsation in nature, the blood may spurt out.
- Venous bleeding: darker in colour than arterial bleeds; usually presents as a slow trickle.
- Capillary bleeding: minor in nature. Infection may be the overriding consideration as a complication in this type of bleed, rather than the bleed itself.

Treatment of severe bleeding: general principles

The general principles for the first aid treatment of severe bleeding are to:

- Put on disposable gloves if available;
- Remove clothing to expose the wound;
- Apply direct pressure to the wound using a sterile dressing if possible or a clean pad; it may be necessary to place further pads;
- If it is not possible to apply direct pressure to the wound, squeeze the edges of the wound together;
- Elevate the wound; raise the injured part of the body above the level of the heart to slow down blood flow to the wound (Figure 14.1);
- Ask the casualty to lie down, with his legs raised if you think that shock may develop;
- Ensure the emergency services are alerted;
- Monitor the casualty's vital signs: observe for signs of shock;
- Keep the casualty warm.

Source: British Heart Foundation (2013)

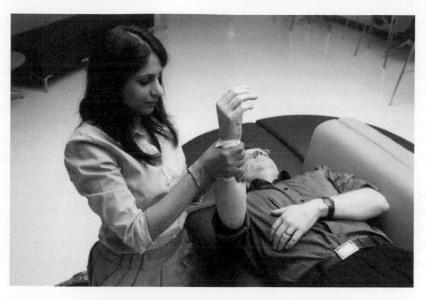

Figure 14.1 Treatment of severe bleeding: if possible, raise the injured part of the body above the level of the heart to slow down blood flow to the wound.

Direct pressure in the form of compressing the wound site will aid clot formation and thus stem the flow of bleeding. Dressing upon dressing should be placed over the wound, until the bleeding stops.

Elevating the limb above the level of the heart is also helpful as gravity will help stem the flow of blood. If this involves the leg, then both legs should be raised. This is easier to manage, and will also assist with the affects of shock.

If bleeding is significant and control is difficult, then the pressure points at the femoral and brachial arteries may be compressed. This is known as indirect pressure, i.e. pressure applied away from the source of bleeding. Indirect pressure should be used in conjunction with direct pressure/compression and elevation.

Epistaxis

Epistaxis (nose bleed) is usually caused by ruptured blood vessels on the nasal septum, close to the Little's area. It is often due to either a blow to the nose or minor trauma, e.g. nose picking, sneezing (St John Ambulance *et al.*, 2011) and can also complicate hypertension and coagulation disorders; in the case of the latter it can be severe and is associated with significant mortality (Wyatt *et al.*, 2012). The recommended treatment is as follows:

- Sit the casualty down, ideally on the floor.
- Ask the casualty to sit upwards and bend forwards at the waist; this will allow the blood to drain from the nostrils; a bowl in front of him allowing blood to drip into it would be helpful.

- Ask the casualty to pinch the nasal alae with the thumb and index finger.
- Encourage the casualty to breathe through his mouth and not his nose.
- Discourage swallowing because this may dislodge the accumulating clot; placing a cork between the casualty's front teeth (Trotter's method) can help to prevent swallowing.
- Also ask the casualty not to speak, cough or spit, again because this may dislodge the accumulating clot.
- After 10 minutes, ask the casualty to release the pressure and re-assess; if the bleeding has not stopped, ask him to re-apply the pressure for another 10 minutes (St John Ambulance *et al.*, 2011); repeat for a third time if necessary.
- If the bleeding stops, encourage the casualty to rest; assess his vital signs; he should be advised not to pick or blow his nose and to avoid hot drinks and spicy foods for at least 24 hours.
- Continued bleeding may require medical attention; if the nose bleed is severe or lasts longer than 30 minutes, take or send the casualty to hospital (St John Ambulance *et al.*, 2011).

MINOR BURNS AND SCALDS

There are approximately 250,000 burn injuries in the United Kingdom every year. The aims of first aid are to stop the burning process, cool the burn, provide pain relief and cover the burn.

- Ensure a safe approach.
- Stop the burning process: remove the heat source and remove burnt clothing (unless it is stuck to the casualty) as soon as possible because it can retain heat. Remove any jewellery, which may become constrictive.
- Cool the burn wound, e.g. cold running tap water for at least 10 minutes (Figure 14.2), this will halt the burning process and reduces pain.
- Cover the burn wound to prevent infection: polyvinyl chloride film (cling film) is ideal in the first aid setting because it is clean, pliable, non-adherent, impermeable and transparent for wound inspection.
- Leave blisters intact – lancing a blister in less than sterile conditions increases the risk of infection.

Source: Allison and Porter (2004); St John Ambulance *et al.* (2011)

POISONING, STINGS AND BITES

Poisoning is usually unintentional, e.g. following exposure to a toxic substance such as carbon monoxide, or can be intentional, e.g. attempted suicide. First aid treatment is usually supportive, particularly with attention to the maintenance

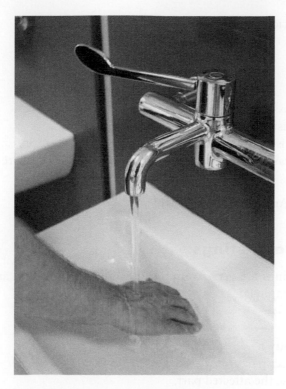

Figure 14.2 Treatment of a severe burn: cold running water for at least 10 minutes.

of a clear airway (altered conscious level is common). In the United Kingdom, insect stings are usually only minor, but occasionally they can cause anaphylaxis. Animal and human bites always require medical attention because of the infection risk.

Alcohol poisoning

Alcohol poisoning is associated with 33% of road traffic accidents, 25% of fatal work-related injuries, 30% of drowning and 50% of burns-related deaths (Wyatt *et al.*, 2012). Complications of alcohol poisoning include:

- respiratory depression;
- cerebral depression;
- peripheral vasodilation leading to heat loss and hypothermia;
- vomit-induced asphyxia.

Signs and symptoms
- Strong smell of alcohol (alcohol bottles/cans evidently).
- Slurred speech.

- Impaired consciousness.
- Flushing.
- Unsteady gait.

Treatment
- Prevent heat loss: cover the casualty with a blanket or a coat.
- Monitor the casualty's vital signs.
- If the casualty is unconscious, place in the recovery position.
- Stay with the casualty until he recovers, or leave him in the care of a responsible adult.

Source: St John Ambulance *et al.* (2011)

Bee and wasp stings

Bee and wasp stings are very painful, can cause local infection and occasionally can cause anaphylaxis.

Treatment
- Help the casualty to sit down.
- Scrape any insect parts off the skin.
- If possible, raise the affected part.
- Apply a cold press or ice to help relieve the pain.
- Advise the casualty to seek medical help if the pain and swelling persists.
- If casualty displays signs of anaphylaxis alert the emergency services; assist him in using his adrenaline auto-injector device if he has one (see Chapter 8).

Source: Jevon (2004)

IMPORTANCE OF RECORD KEEPING

The HSE advice that it is good practice to use a book for recording any incidents involving injuries or illness that dental staff have attended (HSE, 2013). It is advised that the record should include the following:

- Date, time and place of the incident;
- Name and job of the injured or ill person;
- Details of the injury/illness and any first aid administered;
- Outcome: what happened to the casualty immediately afterwards (e.g. went back to work, went home, went to hospital);
- Name and signature of the person dealing with the incident.

Source: HSE (2013)

The above information will help to highlight if there is a trend/pattern to injuries/accidents and can help to possibly identify areas for improvement in the control of health and safety risks.

SUMMARY

This chapter has provided an overview to the principles of first aid in the dental practice. The priorities of first aid have been listed and the responsibilities when providing first aid have been discussed. The assessment of the casualty has been highlighted together with the environmental hazards that may be encountered. The first aid treatment of wounds, severe bleeding, minor burns, scalds, poisoning, stings and bites has been discussed.

REFERENCES

Allison K, Porter K (2004) Consensus on the prehospital approach to burns patient management. *Emergency Medicine Journal*; 21:112–114.

British Heart Foundation (2013) www.bhf.org.uk (accessed 04 October 2013).

Gas Guide (2013) http://www.gas-guide.org.uk/emergencies.html

HSE (2013) *Electrical Injuries,* http://www.hse.gov.uk/electricity/injuries.htm (accessed 04 October 2013).

HSE (2012) *Basic Advice on First Aid at Work,* www.hse.gov.uk (accessed 04 October 2013).

Jevon P (2004) *Emergency Care and First Aid for Nurses: A Practical Guide.* Elsevier, Oxford.

London Fire Brigade (2013) *Emergency Plan,* http://www.london-fire.gov.uk/EmergencyPlan.asp (accessed 24 April 2013).

National Grid (2013) www.nationalgrid.com/uk (accessed 04 October 2013).

St John Ambulance, St Andrew's First Aid & British Red Cross (2011) *First Aid Manual,* Revised 9th edn. Dorling Kindersley, London.

Wyatt J, Illingworth R, Graham C *et al.* (2012) *Oxford Handbook of Emergency Medicine,* 4th edn. Oxford University Press, Oxford.

PRINCIPLES OF FIRST AID IN THE DENTAL PRACTICF

Chapter 15

Professional, ethical and legal issues

Richard Griffith

INTRODUCTION

Law and ethics are now fundamental to the practice of dentistry and underpin your relationship with the profession and with your patients. Probity lies at the heart of your professionalism and requires strict adherence to a code of ethics and the law.

The law informs dentistry at every stage and it is essential that dental professionals understand and are able to critically reflect on the legal issues relevant to practice. This is particularly true in emergency situations when an appropriate and timely response is required.

When dental professionals treat patients they undertake a duty of care towards those persons not to harm them in accordance with the law of negligence. Where dental professionals provide treatment to a patient for a fee then that treatment will be regulated under the laws of contract with the patient able to sue if the contract is not fulfilled. Dental professionals' right to touch a patient will be based on the law of consent and the informed and freely given permission of the patient will be a prerequisite to any lawful treatment. The legal principles of confidentiality and negligence regulate the relationship between the dental professional and the patient while they are in the professional's care.

The standards of the profession and its regulatory body, the General Dental Council, are derived from fundamental human rights principles. These principles largely underpin the law relating to health care and the standards of conduct and performance required of dental professionals by the General Dental Council's *Standards for Dental Professionals* (2005a).

Basic Guide to Medical Emergencies in the Dental Practice, Second Edition. Phil Jevon.
© 2014 John Wiley & Sons, Ltd. Published 2014 by John Wiley & Sons, Ltd.
Companion website: www.wiley.com\go\jevon\medicalemergencies

LEARNING OUTCOMES

At the end of the chapter the reader will be able to:

- Discuss the scope of a dental professional's accountability
- Outline the legal requirements for consent and acting in a patient's best interests
- State the extent of the duty of confidence owed to patients by dental professionals
- Explain the principles of patient safety

THE SCOPE OF A DENTAL PROFESSIONAL'S ACCOUNTABILITY

A registered dental professional is legally and professionally accountable for his or her actions, irrespective of whether they are following the instruction of another or using their own initiative. Healthcare litigation is increasing and patients are increasingly prepared to assert their legal rights. It is perhaps little wonder therefore that the General Dental Council insists that dental professionals are able to practise in accordance with an ethical and legal framework which ensures the primacy of patient and client interest (General Dental Council, 2005a, 2005b).

A thorough and critical appreciation of the legal and professional issues affecting dental practice is essential if you are to develop the professional awareness necessary to satisfy the probity required by the General Dental Council that you are competent to practise as a registered dental professional (see Table 15.1).

Defining accountability

In their seminal work on the subject, Lewis and Batey (1982) defined accountability as 'the fulfilment of a formal obligation to disclose to reverent others the purposes, principles, procedures, relationships, results, income and expenditures for which one has authority'.

An analysis of Lewis and Batey's definition reveals the fundamental nature of accountability. The 'fulfilment of a formal obligation' suggests that accountability has its basis in law. That is, there is a formal or legal relationship between the practitioner and higher authorities (the 'reverent others') that are entitled to hold the dental professional to account. The extent of the scrutiny is illustrated by the inclusion of 'the purposes, principles, procedures, relationships, results, income and expenditures for which one has authority' in the

PROFESSIONAL, ETHICAL AND LEGAL ISSUES

Table 15.1 Advantages of legal awareness for the dental professional

---

The legally aware dental professional:

- *Realises that many aspects of daily life are governed by law*
  Most aspects of life are regulated by law. Legal awareness helps the dental professional appreciate the importance of the legal framework which supports the structure of society.
  It also allows the dental professional to appreciate that personal and social problems may have a legal dimension.

- *Knowingly acts in accordance with legal principles*
  Many parts of the law are necessarily complex and difficult to understand. However, the underlying principles are quite simple. These affect everyone on a day-to-day basis and therefore an understanding of them is important. Indeed, ignorance of the law can bring very serious consequences.

- *Understands the key elements of the legal system*
  Knowledge of the law is of limited value without understanding the various ways in which the legal system works to enforce the law.
  It is important to understand the role of those agencies which have powers to enforce the law and the mechanisms by which the dental professional can seek legal help and advice.

- *Knows when and where to seek appropriate advice*
  The law is vast and constantly changing. The dental professional needs to develop a sense of:
  (a) when the law can help or hinder
  (b) what can be found out and where
  (c) when to seek expert help and
  (d) how to get the appropriate help or advice.

- *Understands the nature of law*
  Even though many day-to-day situations have a legal dimension, there are some problems which the law can do little about, even when in theory this should not be the case.

---

definition. Put more concisely, to be accountable is to be answerable for the acts and omissions within your practice.

This is the approach adopted by the General Dental Council (2005a), the profession's regulatory body, who states in *Standards for Dental Professionals* that:

'You have a professional responsibility to be prepared to justify your actions, and we may ask you to do so. You must be willing and able to show that you are aware of this booklet; and you have followed the principles it explains.

'If you cannot give a satisfactory account of your behaviour or practice in line with the principles explained in this booklet, your registration will be at risk.'

PROFESSIONAL, ETHICAL AND LEGAL ISSUES

Accountability may be defined as being answerable for personal acts or omissions to a higher authority with whom the dental professional has a legal relationship.

Exercising accountability

A common misconception about accountability is that a dentist has some choice over what they are accountable for. Meeting their professional responsibility is often expressed as exercising accountability.

While it is true to say that the General Dental Council sets out the standard of conduct required of dental professionals, accountability cannot be exercised as this would require the practitioner to have control over what they were accountable for. It suggests that dentists can pick and choose whether they wish to be accountable for this action or that patient. This cannot be the case as the purpose of accountability is to protect the public and offer redress to those who have been harmed by dental professionals' acts or omissions. Dental professionals are answerable through the law to a number of higher authorities and it is these higher authorities, not the professionals themselves, who decide if they are to be held to account.

Accountability has four functions as set out in Table 15.2.

Accountable to whom?

Dental professionals owe a formal obligation to answer for their practice to a range of higher authorities. These have a legal relationship with you that enable them to demand that you justify your practice. If you fail to satisfy those requirements, sanctions may be applied against you.

Table 15.2 Functions of accountability

Protective function – The purpose of accountability is to protect the public from the acts or omissions of dental professionals that might cause harm.

Deterrent function – The threat of sanction available to the higher authorities against registered practitioners is seen as protecting the public by deterring acts or omissions that might cause harm.

Regulatory function – By making the dental professional accountable to a range of higher authorities, the law regulates their behaviour and allows action to be taken to protect the public should they breach the regulatory framework.

Educative function – Accountability has an educative function in that those found liable have their cases heard in public with a view to reassuring society that only the highest standards of practice will be tolerated. Other practitioners will learn from such cases and refrain from acting in a similar manner.

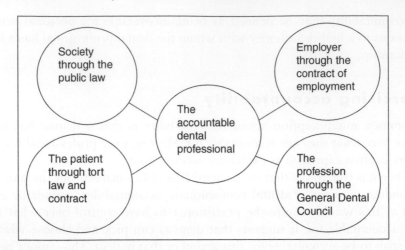

Figure 15.1 Accountability to whom.

In order to provide maximum protection to the public four areas of law are drawn together and can individually or collectively hold you to account. Figure 15.1 depicts to whom you are accountable as a dental professional and the legal basis of that relationship.

Accountability to society

Dental professionals are subject to the same laws as any other member of society. There is nothing about the status of a dentist that exempts them from these laws. If a dentist is suspected of committing a crime during the course of their practice or otherwise they can be called to account.

Accountability to society is achieved through the public law. Many of these laws are derived from Acts of Parliament such as the Road Traffic Act 1988, the Theft Act 1968 or the Offences Against the Person Act 1861. Such Acts are known as public general acts and it is entirely possible to breach them in the course of your practice. A dentist who defrauded the National Health Service (NHS) of £1.4 million, by submitting claims for treating over a hundred patients who were dead and making duplicate claims for others, was jailed for 7 years (Oldham, 2012).

The treatment a dental professional provides to their patient often requires interventions that are personal and intimate in nature. The public law demands that such interventions are only carried out when it is convincingly shown to be medically necessary and by staff who are properly qualified (*R* v *Tabassum*, 2000). Where this occurs the dentist's actions stand outside the criminal law (*Airedale NHS Trust* v *Bland*, 1993). However, the acts of the dental professional will lose their immunity if the necessity cannot be made out or the treatment proceeds without either the consent of a capable patient or the best interests of an incapable patient. For example, a dental practitioner who repeatedly touched a female patient in unnecessary intimate examinations was sentenced to 9 months imprisonment for indecent assault that the judge described as a gross breach of trust (*Yorkshire Evening Post*, 2008).

The public law seeks to protect patients through the regulation of practice and the environment of care. The National Health Service Litigation Authority (2007) estimates that some £500 million is paid annually by the health service in compensation claims and fines for breaching health and safety laws. The cost in human terms can also be high. Mistakes and errors can compromise safety to the point where lives are put at risk and, sadly, fatalities do occur.

To prevent the avoidable loss of life and minimise the days lost to absence, an employer has a legal duty to comply with the requirements relating to health and safety at work. The Health and Safety at Work Act 1974 is the basis of health and safety law in the United Kingdom and it sets out general duties which:

- employers have towards employees and members of the public using their service; and
- employees have to themselves and to each other.

Breaching or failing to comply with these duties are criminal offences.

The employer's general duty is set out in Section 2 of the Health and Safety at Work Act 1974 and states that an employer has a duty to ensure *so far as is reasonably practicable*, the health, safety and welfare at work of employees and any others who may be affected by the undertaking.

The legal standard imposed by the 1974 Act is *reasonably practicable* or *so far as is reasonably practicable*. The standard implies a weighing up of the risk against the cost in terms of time, money or trouble of preventing or controlling the risk.

The duty of employees at work is set out in Section 7 of the Health and Safety at Work Act 1974 that states that:

'It shall be the duty of every employee whilst at work:

- To take reasonable care of their own health and safety and of any other person who may be affected by their acts or omissions; and
- To co-operate with their employer so far as is necessary to enable that employer to meet their requirements with regard to any statutory provisions'.

As well as a duty under the Health and Safety at Work Act 1974 a dental professional is also under a professional duty to act to identify and minimise the risk to patients and clients (General Dental Council, 2005a).

The General Dental Council (2005a) has acknowledged that medical emergencies can occur at any time so all members of staff must know their role in the event of a medical emergency. It is essential therefore that dental professionals and their staff are suitably trained in dealing with emergencies and practise together regularly in simulated emergency situations to maintain their competence. This includes where to locate and use an automated external defibrillator.

A dental professional who raises an issue of health and safety with an employer either directly or through a union is entitled to protection from dismissal and victimisation under the Public Interest Disclosure Act 1998. Under the Act each NHS employer has a duty to establish a procedure for employees to raise concerns where:

- a criminal offence has been, is being or is likely to be committed; or
- the health or safety of an individual has been, is being or is likely to be endangered.

It is essential that employers and staff work together to ensure effective implementation of health and safety measures. This joint approach helps to promote and raise awareness among employers and staff, thereby creating a positive safety culture.

Workplace risk assessments

A risk assessment is the identification of hazards present in the workplace and an estimate of the risk associated with performing the task. A hazard is something that has the potential to cause harm and a risk is the likelihood of that hazard causing an accident or an incident.

There is a legal duty to perform risk assessments under the provisions of the Management of Health and Safety at Work Regulations 1999.

Once a hazard has been identified the likelihood of the risk occurring and the severity of the harm must be considered. The law requires that risks should be reduced *so far as is reasonably practicable*. That means that the degree of risk should be balanced against the time, trouble, cost and physical difficulty of taking measures to avoid it.

On identifying a risk, steps must be taken to minimise it by:

- Elimination of the hazard at source, if this is not possible then the hazard must be reduced;
- If the hazard has to be reduced then action must be taken to control the risk by introducing workplace precautions such as alarms, training and information, safety cabinets, ventilation systems, etc.;
- Once workplace precautions have been introduced then a system to monitor compliance with those precautions must be put in place.

Corporate Manslaughter and Corporate Homicide Act 2007

Under the provisions of this Act dental practices, companies and organisations can be found guilty of corporate manslaughter as a result of serious management failures resulting in a gross breach of a duty of care.

The Act, which came into force on 6 April 2008, clarifies the criminal liabilities of companies including large organisations where serious failures in the management of health and safety result in a fatality.

Dental practitioners can also face gross negligence manslaughter charges where a patient dies as a result of a breach of duty.

A dentist was initially investigated for manslaughter following the death of a child after a general anaesthetic was administered for the extraction of a tooth. The charges were later reduced to five offences under the Health and Safety at Work Act 1974 to which the dentist pleaded guilty. The offences included:

- failure to notify a local hospital that a general anaesthetic was taking place;
- failure to provide the appropriate oxygen monitor;
- failure to provide an assistant for the anaesthetist;
- failure to provide adrenaline in the surgery; and
- failure to estimate the weight of the patient before the operation.

Source: Evans (2001)

Medicines

Modern dental practice often requires the use of medicines in the treatment of patients. While medicines are used for their therapeutic benefits they can and do cause adverse effects in some patients. In *Forman* v *Saroya* (1992) a woman contracted hepatitis as a result of a reaction to halothane anaesthetic administered by her dentist. The dentist ought to have known of her susceptibility because she had suffered a similar reaction when he had given it on a previous occasion. The patient experienced severe abdominal pains soon after the halothane anaesthetic was administered and began to vomit, then suffered lethargy and loss of appetite. These symptoms persisted for just over 2 weeks and required a period in hospital. The dentist was found negligent.

The principal statutory framework for the regulation of medicines are the Human Medicines Regulations (2012). They regulate the licensing, supply and administration of medicines. The Secretary of State for Health has a duty under 2012 regulations to place on prescription only medicines that represent a danger to the patient if their use is not supervised by an appropriate practitioner. Therefore, prescription-only medicines may only be administered by or in accordance with the directions of an appropriate practitioner (Human Medicines Regulations, 2012, reg. 214).

PROFESSIONAL, ETHICAL AND LEGAL ISSUES

Appropriate practitioners include registered dentists who have their own formulary of medicines from which they are authorised to prescribe (Human Medicines Regulations, 2012, reg. 214). Other dental professionals are not appropriate practitioners and generally must only administer medicines in accordance with the directions issued by an appropriate practitioner.

A degree of flexibility over the supply and administration of prescription-only medicines to patients has been provided by the introduction of Patient Group Directions which is a written instruction for the supply or administration of a licensed medicine in an identified clinical situation where the patient may not be individually identified before presenting for treatment.

A Patient Group Direction is drawn up locally by doctors, pharmacists and other health professionals and must meet the legal criteria set out in the Human Medicines Regulations 2012, schedule 16. Patient Group Directions can only be used by registered healthcare professionals acting as named individuals, and a list of individuals named as competent to supply and administer medicines under the direction must be included.

The Human Medicines Regulations 2012, reg. 230 and 232 exempt registered health professionals from the need to obtain a prescription to supply a prescription-only medicine if they act according to a valid Patient Group Direction when assisting a dentist or working in a dental practice in England and Wales.

A Patient Specific Direction is a written instruction for prescription-only medicines to be supplied for administering to a named patient without a prescription. An example would be an instruction by a dentist to supply and administer a medicine in the surgery such as an antibiotic.

To be valid the Patient Specific Direction must:

- be in writing;
- relate to the particular person to whom the medicine is to be administered; and
- be issued by a dentist.

Exemption in an emergency

In an emergency certain prescription-only medicines may be supplied and administered without prescription. The Human Medicines Regulations 2012, reg. 238 allows for the parenteral administration of prescription-only medicines including adrenaline and hydrocortisone injection for the purpose of saving life in an emergency and there is no specific restriction on who is entitled to administer these medicines.

Accountability to the patient

As well as being accountable to society in general, dental professionals are also accountable to the individual patients in their care. The tort or civil law system allows a patient to sue for compensation if they believe that harm has been caused through carelessness. Liability for carelessness is given its legal expression in the law relating to negligence.

Negligence is a civil wrong and best defined as actionable harm. That is, a person sues for compensation because they have been harmed by the carelessness of another person.

Negligence in the healthcare setting has developed under the common law by judges setting rules through decided cases. In certain circumstances, called duty situations, the nature of the relationship between people gives rise to a duty of care. For example, a manufacturer owes a duty to the consumer of his product (*Donoghue* v *Stevenson,* 1932) and one road user owes a duty of care to the other road users in his vicinity (*Rouse* v *Squires,* 1973). Similarly the dentist–patient relationship gives rise to a duty of care (*Kent* v *Griffiths,* 2001). Dentists owe their patients a duty of care and are accountable to the patient if they cause harm by breaching that duty.

In civil law dental professionals are expected to meet the standard of care set by reference to *Bolam* v *Friern HMC* (1957). Known as the Bolam test, it requires that dental professionals meet the standard of the ordinary skilled person exercising and professing to have that special skill or art (*Gold* v *Haringey HA* 1998).

Case law demonstrates that the standard covers the whole of the professional relationship with the patient and includes direct care (*Bayliss* v *Blagg and another,* (1954)), advice giving and record keeping (*Greenfield* v *Irwin (A Firm),* 2001), even the standard of handwriting (*Prendergast* v *Sam and Dee,* 1989). If the dental professional's actions were in keeping with a respected body of professional opinion then practice will not have fallen below the standard required in law and there will be no liability in negligence (*Bolam* v *Friern HMC,* 1957). This will be the case even if there were different ways of performing a task. A judge cannot find negligence just because he prefers one professional's view over another (*Maynard* v *West Midlands RHA,* 1984).

However, in *Bolitho* v *City and Hackney HA* (1997) the House of Lords held that any expert evidence used to support a dentist's actions must stand up to logical analysis. That is, the existence of a common practice does not necessarily mean that it is not negligent. A defendant will not be exonerated because others too are negligent or because common professional practice is slack.

The duty of care to the patient also requires dental professionals to keep their knowledge up to date throughout their career (*Roe* v *Ministry of Health,* 1954).

Emergencies

Dental professionals continue to owe their patient a duty of care in an emergency situation. They are expected to be able to respond effectively to the common emergencies that might arise in dental surgeries. They are expected to ensure that their practice is up to date and evidence based (*Reynolds* v *North Tyneside Health Authority*, 2002).

In relation to treatment decisions taken in an emergency, a dental professional will not be found negligent simply because the reasonably competent dentist would have made a different decision, given more time and information.

In *Wilson* v *Swanson* (1956), the Supreme Court of Canada held that there was no negligence when a surgeon had to make an immediate decision whether to operate during an emergency, when the operation was subsequently found to have been unnecessary.

Moreover, the skill required in the execution of treatment may be somewhat lower because an emergency may overburden the available resources, and, if a dental professional is forced by circumstances to do too many things at once, the fact that he or she does one of them incorrectly would not lightly be taken as negligence.

Carelessness as a crime

Although legal proceedings for carelessness are usually instigated at civil law, it is possible to face criminal prosecution where gross negligence has occurred. In *R* v *Misra and Srivasta* (2004) the Court of Appeal stated that a health professional would be told that grossly negligent treatment which exposed a patient to the risk of death, and caused it, would constitute manslaughter. In this case two doctors refused to call for timely assistance when informed by nurses that a patient was severely ill. The patient died of toxic shock and the doctors were given 14-month suspended jail terms.

Death of a patient in the dental surgery

Where a patient dies in a dental surgery it will likely be an unnatural or sudden death. Such deaths fall into the category that must be reported to the coroner. This includes deaths where:

- the cause of death is unknown;
- the deceased was not seen by the certifying doctor either after death or within the 14 days before death;
- the death was violent or unnatural or suspicious;
- the death may be due to an accident (whenever it occurred);
- the death may be due to self-neglect or neglect by others;
- the death may be due to an industrial disease or related to the deceased's employment;
- the death may be due to an abortion;
- the death occurred during an operation or before recovery from the effects of an anaesthetic;
- the death may be a suicide;
- the death occurred during or shortly after detention in police or prison custody.

It will therefore be necessary to inform the police as well as the emergency medical services of the death. The scene of the death will need to be preserved including the equipment and medicines used so that they can be noted by the police or coroner's officer. Staff involved in the incident should remain available to give a statement for use by the coroner at the inquest.

An inquest heard how a woman died in a dental practice after suffering anaphylactic shock caused by the chlorhexidine in a mouthwash used during the treatment. Staff at the practice failed to recognise that the patient was having an anaphylactic reaction and thought she was having an epileptic fit. The coroner held that only an injection of adrenaline could have saved the patient's life and criticised staff for failing to react in a timely or efficient manner. Protocols were not adhered to and matters, particularly relating to resuscitation, were not done as smoothly as one would have expected from trained professionals (Cockerell, 2011).

Accountability to the employer

An employed dental professional is accountable to their employer through the contract of employment. The contract sets out the terms and conditions of employment and the standard of work expected of the employee (Rideout, 1983). Many of these terms are written in the contract such as salary, holiday entitlement, hours of work, etc. and are known as express contract terms.

In addition many conditions that regulate the relationship between employer and employee are not expressly written into the contract but are there by virtue of decided cases or employment-related legislation. These are known as implied contract terms and include a warranty from the employee to the employer that they will carry out their duties with due care and diligence (*Harmer* v *Cornelius*, (1858)).

Employers are liable for any compensation payable as a result of a civil wrong committed by an employee during the course of their employment, through vicarious liability. Employers will wish to minimise that liability and are entitled under contract law to hold their employees to account through reasonable disciplinary procedures.

For dental professionals, their employer is the most likely authority to hold them to account as a patient with a grievance is more likely to complain to the employer than take legal action. In addition, employment law allows a lower burden of proof when deciding whether an employee is guilty of misconduct.

Unlike criminal law, where the prosecution must prove a case beyond reasonable doubt, or civil law, where a person must show on the balance of probability that a tort was committed against them, employment law only requires that an employer hold an honest and genuine belief that the employee is guilty of misconduct based on the outcome of a reasonable investigation (*British Home Stores Ltd* v *Burchell*, 1980).

Accountability to the profession

Dental professionals are accountable to the profession through the provisions of the Dentists Act 1984 and Health Act 1999, section 60.

The General Dental Council's role is to protect the public by establishing standards of education, training, conduct and performance for dental professionals including all dentists, dental nurses, dental technicians, dental hygienists, dental therapists, clinical dental technicians and orthodontic therapists who must be registered with the council in order to practise.

The General Dental Council is concerned with protecting the public, not dealing with local issues such as a breach of employment contract. Only where the conduct or performance of a dental professional gives rise to concern for public safety will the General Dental Council become involved.

Fitness to practise is the term now used by the General Dental Council to describe a registrant's suitability to be on the register without restrictions. The General Dental Council has the power to hold a registered dental practitioner to account if it is alleged that their fitness to practise is impaired.

The standards by which practitioners are judged, together with the standards the General Dental Council considers the public are entitled to expect, are set out in *Standards for Dental Professionals* (General Dental Council, 2005a). Practitioners who appear before the General Dental Council's fitness to practise panels are held to account against those standards. The standard of conduct and competence expected by the General Dental Council is that of the average practitioner, not the highest possible level of practice. This approach is similar to that adopted by the civil law when judging a skilled practitioner under the Bolam test to determine whether liability in negligence has arisen.

The key difference between negligence law and professional accountability though is that no action in negligence can occur without harm to the patient. However, a breach of the code can occur and a practitioner be held to account even though there has been no harm to a patient.

Strengthening public confidence in the General Dental Council

The General Dental Council is itself regulated by the Council for the Regulation of Healthcare Professionals which oversees the disciplinary decisions of the main bodies of the healthcare professions. It has the power under section 29 of the National Health Service Reform and Health Care Professions Act 2002 to seek a judicial review of a disciplinary decision of a healthcare regulatory body where it considers that decision to be unduly lenient. For example, in *Council for the Regulation of Healthcare Professionals* v *General Dental Council* (2005) the General Dental Council suspended the licence of a dentist to practise for 12 months after he was sentenced to a 3-year community punishment for offences under the Protection of Children Act 1978. The Council for the Regulation of Healthcare Professionals argued that the General Dental Council's sanction in the case was unduly lenient. The court held that a suspension for 12 months was unduly lenient given the serious nature of the offences. The court ordered that in this case removal from the register was the only appropriate penalty.

It can be seen that you are accountable to the profession through the provisions of the Dentist Act 1984 as amended by the Health Act 1999 that empower the General Dental Council to maintain a professional register of dental care practitioners and to determine the standards of education and training necessary to enter the register and to establish standards for practice in order to remain on the register. The standards expected of a registered practitioner are set out in *Standards for Dental Professionals* (General Dental Council, 2005a).

THE FIFTH SPHERE OF ACCOUNTABILITY

All dental practices in England must now be registered with the Care Quality Commission (CQC) and to maintain that registration they must meet the standard for quality and safety set out by the CQC.

The CQC is the regulator for all health and social care services in England including dental practices. They have far reaching powers to take action against practices that fail to meet their standards.

A dental practice was ordered to improve and faced further inspections when CQC inspectors identified major concerns about standards relating to the care and welfare of people who use services, cleanliness and infection control, safety, availability and suitability of equipment, requirements relating to workers, staffing and supporting staff.

The CQC found that the practice did not comply with requirements on cleanliness and infection control. Inspectors could not find evidence to show that denture work was disinfected before fitting. Bags of clinical waste were overfilled and split and stored near clean items, which could have led to cross-contamination.

Inspectors also found that people may have been at risk of harm from equipment that was not fit for purpose with an X-ray machine in poor condition and no device installed to prevent mercury from getting into the waste water system.

There were also insufficient staff with the right knowledge, experience, qualifications and skills, and patients may have been at risk of not having their health needs met.

The poor inspection report led the PCT to remove the dental practice's NHS Contract (Care Quality Commission, 2011).

PROFESSIONAL, ETHICAL AND LEGAL ISSUES

LEGAL REQUIREMENTS FOR CONSENT AND ACTING IN A PATIENT'S BEST INTERESTS

A key requirement of the *Standards for Dental Professionals* concerns respect for patient dignity and choice. Dental professionals are required to:

'Recognise and promote patients' responsibility for making decisions about their bodies, their priorities and their care, making sure you do not take any steps without patients' consent.' (General Dental Council, 2005b at point 2)

Dental professionals need to touch their patients in order to examine or administer treatment or dental care (*F v West Berkshire HA* 1990). The right to touch an individual is limited in law and there is an initial presumption that it must not occur without consent.

The right to self-determination

The law recognises that adults have a right to determine what will be done to their bodies (*Schloendroff* v *Society of New York Hospitals,* 1914). Touching a person without consent will amount to a trespass to the person or, rarely, a criminal assault. Bodily integrity is held in very high regard by the law. Unlike other civil wrongs, such as negligence, that requires harm, any unlawful touching is actionable even if done with the best of motives.

Free choice allows patients to refuse treatment even where this is not in their best interests or might lead to serious health consequences (*Re MB (Caesarean Section),* 1997). As the right to self-determination is held in such high regard it is essential that dental professionals obtain a valid consent from their patients before proceeding with treatment.

Elements of a valid consent

To be a valid defence to a claim of trespass, consent needs to be full, free and reasonably informed.

Full consent

When obtaining consent a patient must agree to all the treatment being proposed (*Williamson* v *East London and City HA,* 1998). Dental professionals must take care to explain all the treatment or touching that will occur when obtaining consent from a patient and ensure that additional treatment or touching is subject to further consent.

Free consent

Consent is an expression of autonomy and must be the free choice of the individual. It cannot be obtained by undue influence (*Re T,* 1992). This does not mean that a dental professional cannot influence a patient's decision. Indeed part of your role is to explain the benefits of treatment to patients in order to obtain consent.

In law, to be undue influence, the action must erode the free will of the patient (*Re U*, 2002). It must be so forceful that the patient excludes all other considerations when making their choice. Undue influence may also be brought to bear by family members. Dental professionals must be certain that the choice being made is that of the patient and not the outside influence of family members (*Re T (Adult: Refusal of Treatment)*, 1992).

Reasonably informed consent

In order to make a free choice a person needs to have sufficient information to inform that choice. For consent to be real, dental professionals are required to explain in general terms what the procedure entails. If a patient can show that the procedure was not explained in broad terms then the consent would be vitiated and liability in trespass would result (*Chatterton v Gerson*, 1981).

As well as a general explanation of the procedure there is also a duty to explain the risks inherent in the procedure. Failing to meet this legal duty will give rise to an action in negligence if the patient was subsequently harmed (*Sidaway v Bethlem Royal Hospital*, 1985).

It can be seen that taking consent is more than accepting the patient's permission. To be a valid consent the decision must be full, free and reasonably informed.

Fraudulent consent

Consent to examination or treatment obtained by fraud will be invalid (*Chatterton v Gerson*, 1981). Such a situation would arise where a dental professional obtained consent for unnecessary treatment from patients.

In *Appleton v Garrett*, (1997) a registered dentist was sued in negligence and trespass for gross overtreatment of patients. The court found that the dentist deliberately embarked on treatment that was unnecessary while deliberately misleading patients as to its necessity because he knew that otherwise they would not have consented to the treatment. The consent was obtained by fraud and was not real and informed consent.

Obtaining consent

Dental professionals may obtain consent in two ways. First, a patient may express their consent. That is, a patient makes known their willingness to be touched. Express consent can be written or oral.

Written consent is usually obtained where a procedure is invasive or perceived as carrying a material risk. A consent form provides a degree of evidential certainty that the patient agreed to treatment. It should not be relied on too heavily, however. A consent form is only as useful as the understanding of the person signing it. When obtaining consent, whether in writing or orally, it is essential that an explanation of treatment and other material facts must be recorded in the patient's file to corroborate the consent.

The second form of consent is an implied consent. This is permission implied through the actions of the patient. A patient opening their mouth when the dental professional asks to examine their teeth is a typical example of an implied consent, as permission to proceed is implied from the action of the patient in response to a request to carry out an examination. It does not mean that agreeing to come to the hospital or surgery implies that a patient agrees to all treatment. Every episode of treatment must be subject to a valid consent.

Consent is a continuous process and may be withdrawn at any time. A withdrawal of consent is as indistinguishable as an initial refusal to consent (*Ciarlariello* v *Schacter,* 1991). Dental professionals must accept that if a patient changes their mind and refuses to continue with treatment then treatment must cease or trespass will occur.

Capacity and self-determination

Capacity in law is the ability to understand and make a balanced decision and is the key to autonomy (*Re T (Adult: Refusal of Treatment)*, 1992). If a person has capacity, dental professionals are bound by their decision. If not, the Mental Capacity Act 2005 can allow another person to make that decision or require the dental professional to determine if the treatment is in their patient's best interests.

Mental Capacity Act 2005

The Mental Capacity Act 2005 sets out a framework for acting for and making decisions on behalf of people aged 16 years and over who lack the mental capacity to make decisions for themselves.

The statutory principles

To underline the Act's fundamental concepts, section 1 establishes a number of statutory principles that must apply to all actions and decisions taken on behalf of a person with incapacity. Dental professionals are required to apply these principles when providing care and treatment for a person who is incapable.

- A person must be assumed to have capacity unless it is established that they lack capacity.

This principle upholds the autonomy of the person. It also means that as the presumption in law is that a person has capacity you do not need to assess the capacity of each patient you see. You are only required to assess capacity where there is a doubt in your mind about a patient's ability to make a decision.

• A person is not to be treated as unable to make a decision unless all practicable steps to help them to do so have been taken without success.

The test for capacity requires a person to understand and use the treatment information given to them. This principle requires you to use simple practical steps to support the person such as a language the person understands, using pictures rather than words, waiting until the person is more alert, etc.

• A person is not to be treated as unable to make a decision merely because they make an unwise decision.

The test for capacity requires that you are able to discern an impairment or disturbance to the person's mind or brain that might be affecting their decision-making ability. Where there is no impairment then you cannot take action under the Mental Capacity Act and must accept the decision as an unwise decision.

• An act done or decision made under this Act for or on behalf of a person who lacks capacity must be done, or made, in their best interests.

Whenever a decision is made on or behalf of a person lacking capacity it must be made in that person's best interests. Where a dental professional believes that a decision maker is not acting in a person's best interests they may challenge that decision. If the conflict cannot be resolved then the Court of Protection can decide what is in the person's best interests.

• Before the act is done, or the decision is made, regard must be had to whether the purpose for which it is needed can be as effectively achieved in a way that is less restrictive of the person's rights and freedom of action.

The Act, for the best of reasons, allows others to interfere in the lives of people who lack capacity. Human rights law allows such interference but only to the extent necessary to achieve a valid objective, such as health care. All actions under the Act must therefore be proportionate to the needs of the individual and all decisions must consider the rights and freedoms of the incapacitated person.

Decision-making capacity

Capacity to make decisions is the key to a person's autonomy and the Act sets out a test for decision-making capacity and the circumstances where a person would be regarded as incapable of making a decision.

The two-stage test

The Mental Capacity Act 2005 sets out a two-stage functional test based on the decision to be made at the time rather than a person's theoretical ability to make decisions generally. The dental professional will need to determine if there is:

(i) An impairment of, or disturbance in, the functioning of the person's mind or brain.
(ii) The extent to which it affects the person's ability to make a decision by assessing whether the person is unable to:
    (a) Understand the information relevant to the decision or
    (b) Retain that information or
    (c) Use or weigh that information as part of the process of making the decision or
    (d) Communicate the decision (whether by talking, using sign language or any other means).

If the dental professional reasonably believes that the person fails any one or more of these four conditions then he or she can conclude that the person lacks capacity for this particular decision.

Designated decision makers

Where a dental professional reasonably believes their patient lacks capacity to decide on treatment then they must consider if a designated decision maker is in place who can consent on the patient's behalf.

The Mental Capacity Act 2005 allows a person to nominate another to make health and welfare decisions for them when they are incapable through a Health and Welfare Lasting Power of Attorney. Dental practices must keep a copy of the registered power of attorney document and ask the attorney for consent before proceeding with treatment in the same way they would ask a patient for consent.

On rare occasions where a person who lacks decision-making capacity has ongoing health and welfare needs, the court can appoint a deputy with power to consent to examination and treatment. Again the dental practice will need a copy of the deputy's authority to give consent, for the patient's records.

Treatment in an emergency

Patients are entitled to make consent to treatment decisions even when an emergency occurs. If the patient has capacity the dental professional must obtain consent before treatment can proceed. A patient can refuse consent even where a medical emergency arises and even where this will have serious consequences on the patient's health.

Where a patient lacks decision-making capacity such as when they are unconscious then the dental professional may act in their best interests out of necessity. Treatment may be given where it is immediately necessary to preserve life or prevent serious harm to the patient (*F* v *West Berkshire HA*, 1990).

Patients can, however, limit the treatment to be provided in an emergency through the use of advance decisions refusing treatment (ADRT).

Advance decisions refusing treatment

This informal instrument can refuse dental treatment in advance. It can also be constructed to refuse life-sustaining treatment. For example, if a patient had a valid and applicable ADRT refusing resuscitation in an emergency then the dental professional would have to respect the wishes of the patient if they were satisfied:

- That the ADRT was in writing;
- Was signed by the maker;
- Was witnessed in the presence of the maker;
- Contained a clear statement as to when it should apply; and
- Contained a statement from the maker stating that it was to apply even if their life was at risk.

Consent and children

Dental professionals will have children under 16 on their case load. In general, the child will be seen with a parent or person with parental responsibility whose consent will be obtained before treatment (see Table 15.3).

The Children Act 1989, Section 2(9) allows a person with parental responsibility to arrange for someone else to exercise it on their behalf.

There is no requirement for this arrangement to be made in writing. For example, children may be brought for treatment by a person without parental responsibility such as a grandparent or childminder. In this situation, as long as the dental professional is satisfied that the person has the authority of someone with parental responsibility, then treatment can proceed with proxy consent.

Some children may seek treatment without their parents being present and dental professionals will need to decide if the child is able to give a valid consent to treatment.

Children reach the age of majority or adulthood at 18. However, while the courts acknowledge that no child under 18 is wholly autonomous, they do recognise the right of a child to consent to medical treatment as they develop and mature with age.

PROFESSIONAL, ETHICAL AND LEGAL ISSUES

Table 15.3 Who has parental responsibility for a child?

Parental responsibility

Parental responsibility is defined as the rights duties, powers duties and responsibilities, which by law a parent has in relation to a child (Children Act 1989, s3)

Mother
Mother has automatic parental responsibility on the birth of the child (Children Act 1989, s2(1) and (2))

Father
Father has parental responsibility if he was married to the child's mother at the time of the birth (Children Act 1989, s2(1))

OR

If he subsequently married the mother of his child (Children Act 1989, s2(3); Family Law Reform Act 1987, s1) OR

If he became registered as the father of the child after 30 December 2003 (Children Act 1989, s4(1)(a)) OR

He and the child's mother make a parental responsibility agreement (Children Act 1989, s4(1)(b)) that is made and recorded in the form prescribed by the Lord Chancellor OR

The Court on his application orders that he shall have parental responsibility (Children Act 1989, s4(1)(c) OR

He obtains a residence order (Children Act 1989, s12 read with s4) OR

He is appointed as the child's guardian and the appointment takes effect (Children Act 1989, s5)

Acquired parental responsibility can only be removed by a Court

Others who can acquire parental responsibility

A person in possession of a residence order which could include the father of the child (Children Act 1989, s12)

A person appointed as the child's guardian once the appointment takes effect; this could include the father of the child (Children Act 1989, s5)

A person, other than a police officer, who is in possession of an emergency protection order (Children Act 1989, s44(4)(c))

A person who has adopted a child (Adoption Act 1976, s12 or Adoption and Children Act 2002, s46)

A Local Authority may additionally acquire parental responsibility

By obtaining a care order (Children Act 1989, s31)

By obtaining a freeing for adoption order (Adoption Act 1976, s18) or a placement order (Adoption and Children Act 2002, s21)

Age however is not the determining factor for decision-making capacity. In law, capacity is based on a person understanding and using treatment information. It is not based on a child reaching puberty.

The Gillick competent child

The issue over whether a child under 16 has the necessary capacity to consent to medical examination and treatment was decided by the House of Lords in *Gillick* v *West Norfolk and Wisbech AHA* (1986) and dental professionals must apply the rule in *Gillick* when determining whether a patient under 16 has capacity to consent to examination and treatment.

When determining whether a child has sufficient maturity and intelligence to make a decision the dental professional will need to take account of:

- the understanding and intelligence of the child;
- their chronological, emotional and mental age;
- their intellectual development; and
- their ability to reach a decision by appraising the advice about treatment in considering the nature, consequences and implications of that treatment (*Gillick* v *West Norfolk and Wisbech AHA* (1986) per Lord Scarman).

The aim of the rule in *Gillick* is to reflect the transition of a child to adulthood. Legal capacity to make decisions is conditional on the child's gradually acquiring the maturity and intelligence to be able to make treatment decisions. The degree of maturity and intelligence needed depends on the gravity of the decision. A relatively young child would have sufficient maturity and intelligence to be capable of consenting to a plaster on a small cut. Equally, a child who had the capacity to consent to dental treatment or the repair of broken bones may lack capacity to consent to more serious treatment (*Re R (A minor) (Wardship Consent to Treatment)*, 1992).

Decision-making capacity therefore does not simply arrive with puberty; it depends on the maturity and intelligence of the child and the seriousness of the treatment decision to be made.

A dental professional must be satisfied that a child has fully understood the nature and consequences of treatment before they can accept their consent or refusal of treatment. It is for the dental professional to decide whether or not a child is Gillick competent and able to consent to treatment. However, the power to decide must not be used as a licence to disregard the wishes of parents whenever the dental professional finds it convenient to do so. Those who behave in such a way would be failing to discharge their professional responsibilities and could expect to be disciplined by their professional body (*Gillick* v *West Norfolk and Wisbech AHA*, 1986).

Where a child is considered Gillick competent then the consent is as effective as that of an adult. This consent cannot be overruled by a parent.

PROFESSIONAL, ETHICAL AND
LEGAL ISSUES

Treating children in an emergency

The same doctrine of necessity applies when treating a child in an emergency as applied to adults under the same circumstances. The Children Act 1989 also allows the dental professional to do what is necessary in the interests of a child's welfare when having care of the child in an emergency (Children Act 1989, Section 3(5)).

DUTY OF CONFIDENCE OWED TO PATIENTS BY DENTAL PROFESSIONALS

Whatever the age of the patient, dental professionals base their treatment on a thorough examination. This includes a personal history where details are disclosed on the basis that the personal information will be kept private and that the dental professional undertakes not to disclose it without permission.

The duty of confidence

There are three key areas that come together to reassure patients that the confidentiality of their health information will be respected.

1. A duty to respect patient confidentiality that is a specific requirement linked to disciplinary procedures in all NHS employment contracts and underpinned by the NHS code of practice on confidentiality (Department of Health, 2003);
2. A legal duty that is derived from case law and supplemented by statute law (*Cornelius* v *De Taranto*, 2001); and
3. A professional duty established by *Standards for Dental Professionals* (General Dental Council, 2005a) and further supplemented by *Principles of Patient Confidentiality* (General Dental Council, 2005b).

The duty of confidence is not, however, absolute. There will be occasions where confidential information about a patient will need to be disclosed to others. Such a disclosure must be to an appropriate person and comply with the requirements of the dental professional's contractual, professional and legal duty of confidence or they will be called to account and face sanction for breaching confidentiality.

It is essential therefore that dental professionals:

- understand the scope of the duty of confidence owed to the patients in their care; and
- disclose information even where given in confidence when it is right and proper to do so.

Contractual duty of confidence

All contracts of employment in the NHS must contain a clause imposing a duty of confidence on all staff that stresses that disciplinary action will result if that duty is breached (Department of Health, 2003). Similar clauses are included in the contracts of dental professionals working in private dental practices.

To discharge this duty, dental professionals will need to show that:

- They will not disclose confidential patient information through inappropriate means such as gossiping;
- When they seek advice about a patient's treatment with a colleague they do so in private so that confidentiality is not inadvertently breached;
- They accurately record information received from and about their patients;
- They keep patient information and records private and physically secure;
- They only access information for the patients in their care; and
- They only disclose patient information to an appropriate source in accordance with the NHS code of practice on confidentiality, the requirements of the law and their code of professional conduct.

The duty extends to all patients, both past and present. Although there is no specific legal or professional requirement that states that a duty of confidence extends to deceased patients, the contractual duty extends confidentiality beyond the grave and includes those who have died.

The professional duty of confidence

The professional requirement for confidentiality is stipulated in the General Dental Council's *Standards for Dental Professionals* (General Dental Council, 2005a).

Clause 3 states that dental professionals must guard against breaches of confidentiality by protecting information from improper disclosure at all times. This imposes a duty not to voluntarily disclose information gained in a professional capacity to a third party. This duty is enforced by the threat of professional discipline.

Confidence and the law

There is a legal obligation to respect patients' confidences that arises out of a general duty on everyone to keep confidential information secret.

A legal obligation of confidence arises when the information:

- Has the necessary quality of confidence; that is, the information is not generally available or known. Information of a personal or intimate nature qualifies (*Stephens* v *Avery*, 1988) and this is largely the type of information dental professionals receive from their patients.

- Has been imparted in circumstances giving rise to an obligation of confidence. In *Attorney General v Guardian Newspapers No 2*, (1988), Lord Keith held that the law has long recognised that particular relationships gave rise to a duty of confidence. One of these was the dentist–patient relationship.
- Has been divulged to a third person without the permission and to the detriment of the person originally communicating the information. An invasion of personal privacy will suffice (*Duchess of Argyll* v *Duke of Argyll*, 1967). As it is in the public interest that medical confidences are kept secret the court will regard an unwarranted disclosure of patient information as detrimental (*Attorney General* v *Guardian Newspapers No 2*, 1988).

The duty of confidence is not absolute

Given the wide scope of the duty of confidence it is perhaps no surprise that dental professionals are reluctant to divulge information about their patients to others. Yet the contractual, professional and legal duties of confidentiality are not absolute and are subject to a range of exceptions that justify disclosure. It is important that dental professionals are aware of these exceptions in order to ensure that information is appropriately disclosed for effective care and protection of vulnerable patients while avoiding a charge of misconduct.

Consent of the patient
Permission to disclose confidential information from the person who originally imparted it is the starting point in law. The courts generally require this consent to disclosure to be in the form of an explicit consent preferably signed by the patient (*Cornelius* v *De Taranto*, 2001). This ruling also reflects the requirements of the Data Protection Act 1998. The consent exception is only valid if the person knows exactly what information is to be disclosed and who is to receive the information.

Disclosure for treatment purposes
Confidentiality can be breached where information is shared with others concerned with the clinical care of the patient. Wide disclosure to any dental professional or doctor is not justified. To require an express consent from a patient each time their case was discussed would be impractical and even detrimental.

Where patients have consented to healthcare, research has consistently shown that they are content for information to be disclosed in order to provide that healthcare (National Health Service Information Authority, 2002).

Disclosing information when specifically asked to do so by a patient
When asked by a patient to pass on confidential information about them then the court regards this as a binding obligation. In *C* v *C* (1946) Justice Lewis

considered the refusal of a sexually transmitted infection clinic to divulge information about a patient despite his request for disclosure. The judge held that, whilst it was important that proper secrecy be observed in sexually transmitted disease clinics, those considerations did not justify a health professional refusing to divulge confidential information to a named person when asked by the patient so to do.

Disclosing information without specific consent

The Department of Health advises that there are a number of exceptions allowing disclosure to appropriate sources without the consent of patient (Department of Health, 2003). These exceptions act as a useful aid when making a judgement about disclosing information concerning a patient.

Where a patient is incapable of receiving information or of consenting to disclosure, then disclosure of care and treatment information to the client's relative or main carer may be judged to be appropriate.

Disclosure to appropriate sources is allowed in cases of suspected abuse of vulnerable adults and children under vulnerable adult and child protection procedures. The public interest in protecting the welfare of children and the vulnerable will outweigh the duty to maintain a confidence (Department of Health, 1999, 2002).

Disclosure in the public interest

The courts accept that when a case concerning disclosure of confidential information comes before them they are required to strike a balance between two competing interests: the public interest in keeping confidential information secret must be weighed against the public interest in allowing disclosure.

The public interest exception covers a broad range of situations including:

- Disclosure in the interests of justice;
- Disclosure for the public good;
- Disclosure to protect a third party; and
- Disclosure to prevent or detect a serious crime.

Disclosure in the interests of justice

A court has the power to order disclosure of confidential matters if it is in the interest of justice and refusing to do so would result in contempt of court. In *Attorney General* v *Mulholland* (1963) two journalists refused to name the sources of information in articles written by them. One of the journalists was sentenced to 6 months and the other to 3 months' imprisonment for contempt.

Dental practitioners, therefore, can be required by the courts to disclose information about their patients both in the form of written statements and in oral evidence where this is necessary in the interests of justice.

Disclosure for the public good

There may be circumstances where the public interest is served by disclosing information even though no crime has been committed or court action taken. This might include disclosing information to the proper authorities about a vulnerable adult or child.

Disclosure to protect a third party

Disclosure of confidential information may be necessary to protect a third party particularly where this concerns a vulnerable adult or child. The dental professional will need to consider the circumstances and use their professional judgement, informed by reference to the common law, to decide if the public interest in protecting the third party outweighs the public interest in keeping confidential information secret.

Disclosure to prevent or detect a serious crime

There may be circumstances when the dental professional is made aware that a patient is a victim of crime or has committed or intends to commit a crime. Before disclosing such information it will be necessary to weigh the seriousness of the crime against the countervailing public interest in maintaining patient confidentiality.

Disclosure is justified where the crime represents a real risk to public safety. That is, there must be a need to prevent or detect a serious crime to justify breaching patient confidentiality as the countervailing public interest in maintaining sensitive health information would generally outweigh disclosure (*W* v *Egdell*, 1990).

Data Protection Act 1998

The Data Protection Act 1998 applies to personal information held on computer or as part of a relevant filing system. This definition would include health records. Under the provisions of the Act a decision to disclose personal health information must be fair and lawful.

To be lawful the disclosure of personal health information must meet the requirements of the common law duty of confidence and be justified (Data Protection Act 1998, Schedules 2 and 3).

Caldicott Guardians

Each NHS organisation has a guardian of person-based clinical information who oversees the arrangements for the use and sharing of clinical information. They ensure that patient-identifiable information is only shared for justified purposes and that only the minimum necessary information is shared in each case.

The Caldicott Guardian plays a key role in ensuring that the NHS satisfies the highest practical standards for handling patient-identifiable information.

The Guardian will actively support work to facilitate and enable lawful and ethical information sharing.

Where a dental professional working in the NHS is unclear about whether a disclosure of information is justified they can seek advice from their Caldicott Guardian.

CONCLUSION

- Law and ethics are now fundamental to the practice of dentistry and underpin the dental practitioner's relationship with the profession and with his or her patients.
- A registered dental professional is legally and professionally accountable for their actions.
- Accountability to society is achieved through the public law that seeks to protect patients through the regulation of practice and the environment of care.
- General Dental Council (2005a) has acknowledged that medical emergencies can occur at any time so all members of staff must know their role in the event of a medical emergency.
- In an emergency certain prescription-only medicines may be supplied and administered without prescription.
- Dental professionals are also accountable to the individual patients in their care through the civil law.
- Dental professionals continue to owe their patient a duty of care in emergency situation and are expected to be able to respond effectively to the common emergencies that might arise in dental surgeries.
- Grossly negligent treatment which exposed a patient to the risk of death, and caused it, would constitute manslaughter.
- Where a patient dies in a dental surgery it will likely be an unnatural or sudden death and such deaths fall into the category that must be reported to the coroner.
- An employed dental professional is accountable to their employer through the contract of employment.
- The standards by which practitioners are judged and the General Dental Council considers the public are entitled to expect are set out in the *Standards for Dental Professionals*.
- A key requirement of the *Standards for Dental Professionals* concerns respect for patient dignity and choice.
- To be a valid defence to a claim of trespass, consent needs to be full, free and reasonably informed.
- Patients are entitled to make consent to treatment decisions even when an emergency occurs.

PROFESSIONAL, ETHICAL AND LEGAL ISSUES

- Where a patient lacks decision-making capacity such as when they are unconscious, then the dental professional may act in their best interests out of necessity where treatment may be given if it is immediately necessary to preserve life or prevent serious harm to the patient.
- If a patient has a valid and applicable ADRT that refuses resuscitation in an emergency, then the dental professional would have to respect the wishes of the patient.
- The same doctrine of necessity applies when treating a child in an emergency as applied to adults under the same circumstances.
- There are three key areas that come together to reassure patients that the confidentiality of their health information will be respected in contract, the law and through the profession.
- The contractual, professional and legal duties of confidentiality are not absolute and are subject to a range of exceptions that justify disclosure.
- It is important that dental professionals are aware of these exceptions in order to ensure that information is appropriately disclosed for effective care and protection of vulnerable patients while avoiding a charge of misconduct.

REFERENCES

Airedale NHS Trust v Bland (1993) AC 789.
Appleton v Garrett (1997) 8 Med LR.
Attorney General v Guardian Newspapers No 2 (1988) 3 WLR 776 (HL).
Attorney General v Mulholland (1963) 2 QB 477.
Bayliss v Blagg and another (1954) 1 BMJ 709.
Bolam v Friern HMC (1957) 1 WLR 582.
Bolitho v City and Hackney HA (1997) 3 WLR 1151.
British Home Stores Ltd v Burchell (1980) ICR 303 (EAT).
Care Quality Commission (2011) *CQC Demands Dental Provider Improves Services.* CQC, London.
C v C (1946) 1 All ER 562.
Chatterton v Gerson (1981) QB 432.
Ciarlariello v Schacter (1991) 2 Med L R 391.
Cockerell J (2011) Woman died after mouthwash reaction. *Press Association* 16 September.
Cornelius v De Taranto (2001) EWCA Civ 1511.
Council for the Regulation of Healthcare Professionals v General Dental Council (2005) EWHC 87.
Department of Health (1999) *Working Together to Safeguard Children.* The Stationery Office, London.
Department of Health (2002) *No Secrets: Guidance on Developing and Implementing Multi-agency Policies and Procedures to Protect Vulnerable Adults from Abuse.* The Stationery Office, London.
Department of Health (2003) *Confidentiality: NHS Code of Practice.* Department of Health, London.

Donoghue v Stevenson (1932) AC 562.

Duchess of Argyll v Duke of Argyll (1967) Ch 302.

Evans N (2001) Cleared dentist faces disciplinary hearing. *This is Lancashire*.

F v West Berkshire HA (1990) 2 AC 1 (HL).

Forman v Saroya (1992) EWHC 13.

General Dental Council (2005a) *Standards for Dental Professionals*. GDC, London.

General Dental Council (2005b) *Principles of Patient Confidentiality*. GDC, London.

Gillick v West Norfolk and Wisbech AHA (1986) AC 112 (HL).

Gold v Haringey HA (1998) QB 481.

Greenfield v Irwin (A Firm) (2001) EWCA Civ 113.

Harmer v Cornelius (1858) 5 CB 236.

Human Medicines Regulations (2012) (SI 2012/1916).

Kent v Griffiths (2001) QB 36 (CA).

Lewis FM, Batey MV (1982) Clarifying autonomy and accountability in nursing services. *Journal of Nursing Administration*; 12(9):13–18.

Maynard v West Midlands RHA (1984) 1 WLR 634 (HL).

National Health Service Information Authority (2002) *Share with Care: Peoples Views on Consent and Confidentiality of Patient Information*. NHSIA, London.

National Health Service Litigation Authority (2007) *Annual Report and Accounts 2007*. NHSLA, London.

Oldham J (2012) *Dentist caged for £1m Fraud*. Birmingham mail; 1.

Prendergast v Sam and Dee (1989) 1 Med LR 36.

R v Misra and Srivasta (2004) EWCA Crim 2375.

R v Tabassum (2000) 2 Cr App R 328.

Re MB (Caesarean Section) (1997) 2 FLR 426.

Re R (A minor) (Wardship Consent to Treatment) (1992) Fam 11.

Re T (Adult: Refusal of Treatment) (1992) 3 WLR.

Re U (2002) Lloyd's Rep Med 93.

Reynolds v North Tyneside Health Authority (2002) Lloyd's Rep Med 459.

Rideout RW (1983) *Principles of Labour Law*, 4th edn. Sweet & Maxwell, London.

Roe v Ministry of Health (1954) 2 QB 66 (CA).

Rouse v Squires (1973) 2 All ER 903.

Schloendroff v Society of New York Hospitals (1914) 211 NY 125.

Sidaway v Bethlem Royal Hospital (1985) AC 871.

Stephens v Avery (1988) Ch 449.

W v Egdell (1990) 2 WLR 471.

Williamson v East London & City HA (1998) Lloyd's Rep Med

Wilson v Swanson (1956) 5 DLR (2d) 113 (Canadian Supreme Court).

Yorkshire Evening Post (2008) Leeds dentist jailed for groping patient. *Yorkshire Evening Post*; 1 April 2008: p. 1.

PROFESSIONAL, ETHICAL AND
LEGAL ISSUES

Index

ABCDE assessment, 6–7, 26–47
  for altered level of consciousness, 97
  principles of, 28
abdominal thrusts *vs.* chest thrusts, 149–50
acute illness, clinical signs of, 27
adhesive pad electrodes, 154
adrenaline, 176
  for anaphylaxis, 111–12
  drugs used in dental practice, 177
  mode of action, 176
  pre-filled syringe, 176
adrenaline auto-injector device, 112–13
adrenal insufficiency, 85–6
  causes of, 85–6
  clinical features of, 86
  treatment of, 86
adult pocket mask, 166
AED, 19
airway, assessment of, 29–30
airway equipment, 16–17
airway management, 131–51
airway obstruction
  causes of, 132
  complete, 132
  partial, 132
  recognition of, 132
  treatment of, 30
allergies, 8
altered level of consciousness, 96–7
  ABCDE approach for, 97
  causes of, 96

investigations of, 96
treatment of, 97
ambulance, calling 999 for, 10–11, 83, 92
ambulance control centre, 10
ampoules, 178
anaphylaxis, 104–16
  causes of, 106–7
  clinical features of, 107–9
  definition of, 105
  diagnosis of, 107–9
  incidence of, 105
  pathophysiology of, 105
  risk assessment in, 113–4
  treatment of, 109–13
angina, 8, 67–9
  precipitants of, 67
  signs and symptoms of, 67
  treatment of, 68–9
angioedema, 108
Aspirin, 82
  indication 179
  mode of action, 179
  paediatric doses, 179
  presentation, 179
  side effects, 179
asthma, 8, 49–55
  causes of, 49–50
  hospital admission, indications for, 53
  incidence, 49
  life-threatening, signs of, 50, 54
  pathogenesis, 49
  poor outcome, factors for, 55

Basic Guide to Medical Emergencies in the Dental Practice, Second Edition. Phil Jevon.
© 2014 John Wiley & Sons, Ltd. Published 2014 by John Wiley & Sons, Ltd.
Companion website: www.wiley.com\go\jevon\medicalemergencies

asthma, *(Continued)*
  signs and symptoms of, 50, 54
  treatment of, 50–53
auto-injector devices, 178
automated blood pressure devices, 44
automated external defibrillation
    algorithm, 118, 119
automated external defibrillator
    (AED), 19, 152
  in cardiopulmonary resuscitation, 124–6
  checking of, 21–2
AVPU scale, 33

bag-mask ventilation, 143–7
  in dental chair, 145–7
  on floor, 144–5
  gastric inflation with, 147
  ineffective, 147
barrier devices, 139
bee and wasp stings, 200
beta-2 adrenergic stimulant, 185
blood glucose, measurement of, 83–5
  indications for, 84
  procedure for, 84–5
blood glucose measurement device, 20, 83–5
blood pressure, measurement of, 41–4
  arm selection for, 41
  automated devices for, 44
  errors in, 44
  Korotkoff sounds, 41
  manual, 42–3
  systolic and diastolic, 41
breath-actuated inhalers, 58
breathing
  assessment of, 30–31
  treatment of, 31–2
breathing equipment, 17–18
bronchospasm, 132
Buccolam, 182
burns and scalds, 200

cardiac arrest, 2
  in dental chair, 9
  on floor, 9
  in toilet, 9
  in waiting room, 9
cardiopulmonary resuscitation
    (CPR), 8–9, 117–30
  AED in, 124–6
  chest compressions, 122–3, 126–9
  in dental chair, 9, 118–26
  on floor, 9, 127
  procedure for, 118–26
  responsiveness, assessment of, 120–21
  safer handling, 8–9, 126–7
cardiovascular disease (CVD), 66–77
  angina, 67–9
  myocardial infarction, 69–73
  palpitations, 73
  syncope, 74–6
cerebral haemorrhage, 94.
    See also stroke
cerebral infarction, 94.
    See also stroke
chain of survival, 2
checking equipment, 20–3
chest compressions, 126–9. *See also*
    cardiopulmonary resuscitation
    (CPR)
  in dental chair, 126–7
  on floor, 127, 128
  safer handling during, 126–7
  techniques for, 127–9
chest thrusts *vs.* abdominal thrusts, 149–50
choking, 147–50
chronic obstructive pulmonary
    disease (COPD), 56–7
  causes of, 56
  clinical features of, 57
  incidence, 56
  treatment of, 57
circulation
  assessment of, 32–3
  treatment of, 33

circulation equipment, 18–19
compromised breathing, treatment
    of, 31–2
COPD, 56–7

defibrillation, defined, 152
dental practitioners, 211
dental professional's accountability
    accountability to employer, 215
    accountability to profession, 216
    carelessness, 214
    contractual duty of confidence,
        227
    decision-making capacity, 221
    defining, 205–6
    disclosure in the public interest,
        229–31
    duty of confidence, 226
    emergencies, 213–4
    exercising, 207–8
    fifth sphere of, 217
    Gillick competent child, 225
    introduction, 204
    legal requirements, 218
    Manslaughter and Corporate
        Homicide Act, 211–2
    obtain consent, 219–20
    professional duty of confidence,
        227–8
    scope of, 205
    to society, 208
    the two-stage test, 222
    treatment decisions, 223
dentures, 135
diabetes, 8
diastolic blood pressure, 41
disability, assessment of, 33–34
displaced tongue, 132
drugs, recommended, 19
dry powder inhalers, 58

ECG interpretation skills, 152
endocrine disorders, 78–87
    adrenal insufficiency, 85–6
    hypoglycaemia, 78–83

epilepsy, 8
EpiPen, 113
epistaxis, 199–200
equipment inventory, 20
exposure, 34
external defibrillation, automated,
        152–8
    factors affects, 154
    implantable cardioverter
        defibrillator, 157–8
    introduction, 152–3
    physiology of, 153
    procedure for automated, 155–8
    safety issues, 158
    transthoracic impedance, 154
    ventricular fibrillation, 153

FBAO treatment of, 172, 174
finger sweep, 150
first aid in dental practices
    assessment of the casualty, 190–91
    casualty's clothing, 193–4
    environmental hazards, 191
    low-voltage electricity, 192
    priorities of, 190
    responsibilities when, 190
foreign body airway obstruction
        (choking), 147–50. See also
        airway obstruction
    follow-up in, 150
    incidence of, 147
    recognition of, 147–8
    treatment procedure for, 148–50

The General Dental Council, 204,
        210, 216
glucagon, 81–2
    dose and route of administration,
        180–81
    indications, 180
    mode of action, 180
    presentation, 180
    side effects, 181
GlucoGel, 81
glucometer, 84

glyceryl trinitrate (GTN)
    indications, 181
    mode of action, 181
    paediatric doses, 182
    presentation, 181–2
    side effects, 182
    spray, 68
gurgling, 29

head tilt, chin lift, 133, 140
history taking, 7
HSE advice, 202
human factors and teamwork, 11–12
hyperventilation, 55–6
hypoglycaemia, 78–83, 185
    causes of, 79–80
    clinical features of, 80
    diagnosis of, 80
    incidence of, 79
    risks associated with, 79
    treatment of, 80–3
hypotension, 27

implantable cardioverter defibrillator
        (ICD), 155
inhaled beta-2 agonist, 113
inhaler, 52, 57–61
    drug delivery using, 59
    drugs administered using, 58
    procedure for, 59–61
    types of, 58

jaw thrust, 134

Korotkoff sounds, 53

laryngeal oedema, 132

manual defibrillator, checking of,
        21–2
medical emergencies
    in dental practice poster, 44–6
    General Dental Council guidelines
        on, 4–5
    incidence of, 3–4

medical problems, existing, 8
The Mental Capacity Act 2005, 220
mercury sphygmomanometer, 42
midazolam, 182
    buccal administration of, 91
    dose and route of administration,
        184
    indications, 184
    mode of action, 183
    paediatric doses, 184
    presentation, 183
    side effects, 184
mouth-to-mask ventilation, 141–3
    in dental chair, 143
    on floor, 142
    pocket masks for, 141–2
mouth-to-mouth ventilation, 139–41
    barrier devices, 139
    gastric inflation with, 141
    procedure for, 139–40
    rescue breaths, ineffective, 141
myocardial infarction (MI), 69–73
    pathogenesis of, 69–70
    signs and symptoms, 70–71
    treatment of, 71–3

National Institute for Clinical
        Excellence (NICE), 89
neuroglycopenia, 80
neurological disorders, 88–103
    altered level of consciousness, 96–7
    recovery position, placing patient
        in, 97–101
    spinal injury, 101
    stroke, 93–6
    tonic–clonic seizure, generalised,
        88–93
non-rebreather mask, 161

open and clear airway, techniques to,
        133–5
    dentures, 135
    head tilt, chin lift manoeuvre, 133
    jaw thrust manoeuvre, 134
    suction, 134–5

oral glucose solution/tablets/gel/
    powder
  indication, 185
  presentation, 185
oropharyngeal airways, 16
  cautions during use of, 136
  correct size of, estimation of, 136
  insertion of, 136–8
  use of, 135–8
oxygen, administration of, 38–40
oxygen cylinders, 23–5
oxygen face mask with tubing, 18

paediatric AED pads, 169
paediatric emergencies, 160–73
  ABCDE assessment of child
  airway management, 161, 164–65
  breathing, 162
  circulation, 162
  disability, 162
  face masks, 166
  management of, 170–71
  modifications to, 163–64
  principles of paediatric
    resuscitation, 162–63
  principles of performing chest
    compressions, 167–68
  priorities of resuscitation, 163
  recovery position, 170
  Resuscitation Council (UK), adult
    choking guidelines, 171–72
  use of, 168–70
  ventilations, 165
paediatric face masks, 166
paediatric pocket mask, 167
Paediatric use marketing
    authorisation (PUMA), 182
palpitations, 73
panic attack, 109
pMDI, 58
pocket mask, with oxygen port, 17
poisoning, stings and bites, 200
  alcohol poisoning, 200–201
  record keeping, 202–3
portable suction device, 16

pressurized metered dose inhaler
    (pMDI), 58
Principles of Dental Team Working,
    5
pulmonary oedema, 132
pulse oximeter, 34
pulse oximetry
  advantages of, 36
  complications of, 38
  limitations of, 37
  mechanics of, 35–6
  oxygen saturation, normal range
    for, 36
  principles of, 34–8
  procedure for, 36–7
  role of, 35
  uses of, 36

recovery position, 97–101
  complications, 101
  indications for, 98
  procedure for, 98–101
  safer handling during, 101
  variations of, 98
respiratory disorders, 48–65
  asthma, 8, 49–55. *See also* asthma
  chronic obstructive pulmonary
    disease, 56–7
  hyperventilation, 55–6
respiratory rate indicator, 40
resuscitation bag, 20
Resuscitation Council (UK), 171
Resuscitation Council (UK)
    Standards, 5–6
resuscitation equipment, 15–25
  checking of, 20–23
  overview, 15
  recommended, 16–20
resuscitation training, 1
risk assessment, medical, 7–8

safer handling, 8–9
Salbutamol (ventolin), 185–6
  dose, 187
  mode of action, 186

Salbutamol (ventolin), *(Continued)*
  side effects, 187
  suggested procedure, 186
self-inflating bag, 21, 123, 144
self-inflating resuscitation bag,
    checking of, 21
short-acting beta-2 adrenoceptor
    stimulant inhaler, 52
snoring, 29
spacer device, 53, 61–4
  advantages of, 61–2
  indications for, 62
  principles of, 62
  procedure, 62–4
  types of, 61
spinal injury, 101
standards for dental professionals, 4–5
sterile needles, 19
sterile syringes, 18
stridor, 29
stroke, 93–6
  FAST approach for, 94, 95
  pathogenesis, 94
  symptoms of, 94
  treatment of, 94–6
suction, 134–5
syncope, 74–6
  causes of, 74–5
  signs and symptoms of, 75
  treatment of, 75–6
systolic blood pressure, 41

tachycardia, 27
tachypnoea, 27
team leader, attributes of, 12
tonic–clonic seizure, generalised,
    88–93
  ambulance, call 999 for, 92
  causes of, 90
  observations during, 92–3
  personalized care plane, 93
  signs and symptoms of, 89
  treatment of, 90–92

urticaria, 107, 108

vagal manoeuvre, 75
vasovagal, 74
vasovagal attack, 109
ventilations, 138–47, 165
  bag-mask ventilation,
    143–7
  mouth-to-mask ventilation,
    141–3
  mouth-to-mouth ventilation,
    139–41

wheeze, 30
wounds and bleeding
  categories of, 198
  principles of, 196
  treatment, 199
  types of, 195–6

Printed and bound by CPI Group (UK) Ltd, Croydon, CR0 4YY

09/10/2024

14571429-0004